Help! I am a Christian, Why am I Sick?

Help! I am a Christian, Why am I Sick?

Klay E. Rogers

Help! I am A Christian, Why Am I Sick?

Published by Aspire Publishing Group

For information:
Aspire Publishing Group
5435 N. Garland Ave., Ste 140, LB 138
Garland, Texas 75040

E Mail: KlayCPA@MSN.com
WWW:AspirePublishingGroup.com

For speaking engagements contact
Aspire Publishing Group
E mail@ KlayCPA@MSN.Com

ISBN-13: 978-0-9792535-0-8
ISBN-10: 0-9792535-0-0

Printed in the United States of America

In Memory of

Teresa Ann Rogers

February 22, 1966 – March 13, 2004

Oh What Joy (Teresa's Song)

Lyrics by Klay Rogers ~ Music by Brent Rogers

(The song can be heard at www.KlayRogersCPA.com/personal/index.html)

I looked at you to ask, "Are those natural curls?"
You have a glow I cannot tame.
Ice blue eyes that see deep into my world.
I love your tall and slender frame.

Chorus

I found the peace and oneness that I always had longed for.
I have the peace and oneness to always enjoy.
I'm blessed beyond my great imagination.
I married an angel from heaven, oh what joy.

A mother's hand to mold the child for our Lord.
Your perseverance through despair.
Making the baby laugh with a song and your touch.
You give a kiss to say I care.

Chorus

Your nature is sweetness and your heart is pure.
An excellent wife, who can find?
Never calling attention to yourself.
With serving the Lord first on your mind.

Chorus

Contents

Acknowledgements

I want to thank everyone who supported Teresa during her illness. This includes the wonderful doctors Dr. Virginia Stark-Vance and Dr. Edward Gilbert and their wonderful staffs. There was a great circle of friends from Nortel Networks in Richardson, Texas, and Raleigh, North Carolina (Kim, Karen, Richard, Curt, Don, Jacqui, to name a few). I thank the loving church family at Gateway Community Church in Wylie, Texas, and Pastor Blake Switzer and the attentive staff at Pleasant Valley Church in Thomaston, Georgia. I also thank the friends in my neighborhood (Joel and Cathy, Alan and Kelly, Joe and Linda, Robert and Mary, Troy and Lesly, Lynn and Lynne, Val, and many others) and my extended circle of friends (Scott and Connie, John R., Pastor Terry Sutton, Pastor Jerry Wilson and his family, Carla and Lindy, Marty B., Terri C. and others). I thank my theological editor, Rick Wade of Garland, Texas, and literary editor William Greenleaf (www.williamgreenleaf.com), of Port Angeles, Washington, whose expertise has raised the level of this book's content in all areas. And finally I thank my family: my father, Stan Rogers, and his wife, Pat, my very musically gifted younger brother, Brent Rogers, who has a big heart, and my wonderful kids, Ashley, Brandon and Blake.

Introduction

Disease is a complex subject. I decided to write this book because, when disease touched my life, I felt lost as I sought answers from a broad community of believers. If you're like me, maybe you've wondered why the Lord would allow you or someone you love to be touched by disease.

I write as a layman in the church, not as a scholarly theologian or a medical professional. The opinions and testimony in this book are those of a man who has searched firsthand for answers to the difficult questions surrounding this subject. If you have a disease, it may take some time for you to fully understand your situation. Yet with knowledge comes freedom and peace. It is my hope that by reading this book you will find peace in your circumstance. I believe that the Lord heals people every day. However, this book will not offer you promises beyond what Scripture makes clear.

One day in September 2001, my wife, Teresa, came down with a migraine headache. Since she had a history of migraines, her symptoms did not initially alarm us. She took her normal medicine, but after a few days, the pain did not subside. Her doctor prescribed a new medication, but it didn't help either. On September 13, 2001, two days after the New York City bombings, Teresa stopped eating. I became very concerned and decided it was time to go to the emergency room of our local hospital.

There, the doctors performed a CT scan and gave us the bad news. There was a mass in the right frontal lobe of her brain, and surgery would be necessary within the next few days. Based on every preliminary indicator, it looked like the most common kind of brain cancer, called glioblastoma multiforme (GBM). All GBMs are grade four; they can double in size in ten days and have only a 2% survival rate after five years. There is no known cure. In the United States, GBMs affect over 18,000 people each year.

My initial reaction was denial. It couldn't be true! Teresa was thirty-six years old at the time, and the sweetest and most loving person you would ever meet. She had grown to become a beautiful Christian woman. We had three children and had been married for fourteen years. She had a successful job at an international telecommunications company. If the news about the cancer were true, we would fight with all our energy and become part of the 2% who survived.

Within the next few days, we met with the neurosurgeon and the neuro-oncologist to understand the disease, the risks, and the treatment procedures. They performed a craniotomy and did their best to remove the mass of cancer cells. The biopsy confirmed that it was GBM. We began the most complex of treatment programs, which included chemotherapy, radiation, and dissolvable wafers left in the brain after surgery. I added a nutritional treatment program and some alternative medical treatments that did not conflict with the allopathic recommendations.

Teresa recovered from the surgery with amazing success. She experienced none of the usual side effects: no paralysis, change in personality, headaches, or post-operative complications, such as swelling or bleeding. The medical professionals were very pleased with the results. For the next eleven months, Teresa underwent various treatments, beginning with conforming field radiation and followed by a rotating protocol of chemotherapies prescribed by the renowned Dr. Henry Friedman of Duke University Medical Center in Raleigh, North Carolina. The typical GBM patient has recurrence within a year, which often requires a second craniotomy. Teresa, by contrast, reached the one-year mark in perfect health. In fact, she discontinued treatments and outperformed all expectations for twenty-four months.

In the twenty-fifth month, she had recurrence. The cancer was in a new location, still on the right side, but this time deep in the white matter of the brain at about ear level. Surgery was not an option without severe consequences. She started chemotherapy treatments again, but they were ineffective. Over the next three months, she received three completely different drugs with three completely different delivery modes. None of them had any impact on the cancer cell growth. GBM is known as a "smart cancer" because the cells can mutate and become resistant to the prescribed treatments. The cancer grew without restraint.

In spite of all our prayers, Teresa died on March 13, 2004, at the age of thirty-eight. Her death was peaceful. She did not experience any pain and died rather quickly, without the anticipated coma. We were all with her till the end, and she knew she was greatly loved. We had closure and had been able to say everything that needed to be said. The Lord had approved her home-going, and she received it as an obedient servant. She ran her race and finished well. Teresa is now in the presence of the Lord, experiencing an indescribable feeling of freedom, wholeness, and peace, and she does not want to return to this life.

This was the most difficult trial of my life. I sought the Lord on my knees and pleaded with Him to heal Teresa. Those of you who are facing disease may understand the way I felt. I spent hours reading on the Internet and woke up countless times at night thinking about the situation. I had hours of conversation with health-care professionals. I also sought counsel from my community of fellow believers, who belonged to many churches and different denominations. They showered us with love and compassion beyond our greatest expectations.

However, among the community of believers I found a distinct lack of knowledge and training in medical matters, which left little possibility of a substantial biblically-based response that could lead to healing. We were offered sincere yet simplistic answers, such as, "God will heal you if he wants to," and "God has a purpose." It was this gap in spiritual training that prompted me to write this book. As stated in Hosea 4:6, "My people are destroyed for lack of knowledge." Yes, lack of knowledge is devastating and keeps us from the blessings of God.

My primary goal is to prevent disease before it occurs. My secondary goal is to have a solid biblical response to disease when it does occur. I have observed that the body of Christ worldwide is not trained to respond to disease, and that Satan is having his way. I have asked a thousand questions: Why are some people healed and some are not? Is it true that healing was more common in biblical times than today, and if so, why? Healings seem so arbitrary, almost like a lottery. Does God have a logical plan or criteria as to who gets healed and who does not? Are the healings we see on television valid? Does anyone go back and talk to the healed a year later to see if their situation was temporary or permanent? Did the healing accompany a change of heart in that person, or a new spiritual revelation?

Sometimes it seems as if we have become so smart that we don't need God. I would say that most pastors and church leaders consider themselves to be only indirectly responsible for the physical health of their flock, and therefore they avoid teaching on this subject. Conversely, medical doctors don't pastor. There is therefore a great void where those two professions meet. In the alternative medical community, on the other hand, the clear majority of holistic practitioners are not operating within biblical guidelines. In my experience, the typical holistic health-care practitioner is more inclined to speak New Age philosophy than biblical truth. I have learned to distinguish the holistic approach to disease from what I refer to as a "biblically holistic" approach. The two are very different.

I want to emphasize my primary motivation for writing this book. There is little possibility of finding a ministry to meet our needs when there is such a lack of knowledge within the church about medical information and scriptures that are relevant to our physical health. Typically, the church leadership, for various reasons, does not take responsibility for the physical health of their flock. I hope that this book can help church leaders to become more confident addressing believers' physical health through effective teaching and ministry.

There is almost always a connection between the spiritual health of the saints and their physical health.

Throughout this book, I will demonstrate that there is almost always a connection between spiritual health and physical health. The biblical directives of our heavenly Father are not only spiritual in purpose. When He says, "Don't be anxious," "Forgive one another" (i.e. do not be bitter), and "Do not fear," He has in mind our physical well-being in addition to our spiritual well-being.

As you read this book, I ask two things of you. First, if you're fighting a disease, realize that your battle is physical *and spiritual.* Satan does not like to be exposed, and he'll give you a thousand reasons not to read your Bible, to receive encouragement from others, or to be encouraged by reading this book. I encourage you to be persistent, to resist him, and to keep reading—but of course, don't substitute this book for the time you spend in God's Word. Second, because this topic is complex, read the *entire* book so that you won't draw the wrong conclusions. I've seen it happen before. If you only read two chapters, you'll likely miss the primary message. I realize that we may disagree on some issues, but I think you'll agree with the primary message once you understand it.

Chapters 2, 3, and 4 examine different and seemingly unrelated aspects of disease in our lives. I call them "puzzle pieces 1, 2, and 3." It won't be until chapter 5, when the three pieces are put together, that you'll be able to see the whole picture. Then the full scheme of Satan will be revealed.

CHAPTER 1

BIBLICAL EXPLANATIONS FOR DISEASE

In America, we are conditioned into simplistic "step 1-2-3" problem-solving. For example, if my problem is hunger, I immediately have a solution: find the next drive-thru and get something to eat. "What is your pleasure—chicken, tacos, or a hamburger?" The problem is solved in less than ten minutes.

Then there are more serious examples of simplistic thinking. "Oh, so you have cancer? Obviously you did something wrong somewhere in step 1, 2, or 3. Therefore, you should take a couple of pills and maybe a vitamin or two, and the cancer will go away. In a few days, everything should be fine." This type of thinking could not be further from the truth. It never addresses the root problem that caused the situation in the first place.

The topic of healing clearly polarizes the church. A majority on one end of the spectrum don't believe that God necessarily heals today. A minority on the opposite end believe that the gift of healing is active and that most everyone should be healed here on earth. Even fewer people in the middle recognize that God does heal, although they do not necessarily have a scriptural explanation for how or when it occurs or how to respond to disease. Many in the worldwide church explain disease this way: "It's the perfect will of God that you should never be sick. Therefore, if you're sick, it's obvious that you have a sin issue in your life. After all, it's right there in James 5:16: 'Confess your sins so that you may be healed.'" Then there are those who are so offended by the notion that sin might have caused their disease that they won't even talk to the people in the other group, going so far as to question their salvation! I've heard it said, "If they can't get the healing verses right, can they be trusted with the basic plan of salvation?"

> *The topic of health and healing clearly polarizes the church.*

I am convinced that when we stand before the throne of the Lord, we will *all* discover that our theology is wrong somewhere. In my place as a layman in the church, I'm not comfortable with any of these schools of thought. I prefer to keep an open mind with a full helping of humility on the various disputed issues. You will better understand my perspective as you read.

I have found at least seven explanations for disease in Scripture. I will summarize them here and develop them more fully later in this chapter. The problem I've experienced in the past is that the student of God's Word will become distracted by a minor issue and then fail to understand the central issue. You may not agree with some of my observations, but that doesn't mean my primary message is incorrect. As previously stated, I will summarize my message in chapter 5.

Scriptural explanations for diseases include:

- *The wrath of God.* In some instances, disease falls on people because God is angry and desires to bring about a change in the situation.

- *The sins of others* bring disease upon people.

- *The sins of our ancestral fathers* bring disease upon people. This explains some of the diseases of children. In this situation, we may not be the cause of disease. However, we still bear responsibility in our *response* to the disease. Scripture gives an example of that response; I will point out the scriptures later in this chapter.

- We have disease *because of our own sin.* This is complex, so I ask you to read the entire book before forming a judgment. As saints who are secure in our salvation, we are free from the penalty of sin. However, there are still consequences to sin in this life, and this might be a disease.

- A disease *serves the purpose of God.* This is often a mystery to us. I don't believe that we will fully understand how God makes "all things work together for good," even through disease, until we stand in His presence. However, disease does serve His purpose in some situations.

- Sometimes God uses disease *to call us home.* Plain and simple, we don't live forever on this earth. We must die, and sometimes death occurs because of disease.

- There can be a *combination* of any of the above reasons.

I also recognize that, in this day and age, environmental poisons can put us at risk of disease. I could list environmental poisons as an eighth reason, but I can't give you a scriptural basis for it. However, I will give you three real-life examples.

In 1998, my mother was ill with liver cancer and received treatment from American doctors in a hospital located in Mexico just south of San Diego. The doctors in that hospital believed that there was a correlation between the cancer rates in various U.S. cities and the quantity of chlorine in the water. As a second example, take a look at the warning notices on packages of toothpaste that contain fluoride, instructing the consumer to contact medical help or a poison control center immediately if more than a toothbrush amount is swallowed. Fluoride and chlorine are poison in their undiluted forms.

A third example is the chemical *dioxin,* a term used to describe over a hundred chemicals, which is released when plastic is either heated or frozen. For example, plastic containers and wraps that are heated in the microwave can produce and transfer poisonous toxins into the food. Plastic containers in the freezer can produce dioxin and transfer it into the food or water. Glass containers are better suited for use in the microwave or freezer. One form of dioxin has been tied to breast cancer, but nevertheless, the entire chemical group is carcinogenic.

These and similar poisons can lead to serious diseases. However, because they are not mentioned in the Scriptures, they are not within the scope of my study. (I recommend an excellent book that includes a chapter on the subject of environmental hazards: *Super Health: 7 Golden Keys to Unlock Lifelong Vitality*, by K.C. Craichy.) Wars, accidents, and murders were not given as reasons for disease, per se. Plagues are considered a disease and can be explained in some situations by Scripture. My list of seven should cover almost every reason for disease affecting the church today.

I don't know if any research has been conducted to determine the most common spiritual root causes of disease. Nevertheless, it's my opinion that most diseases facing the saints today are caused by our own sin issues on some level. Diseases we have inherited from our generational fathers are likely the second leading cause, and the other causes account for the rest.

I have dedicated most of this book to exploring three reasons for disease: our own sin issues, our response to disease resulting from the sin of our ancestral fathers, and the sin of others. These are the only scenarios to which we may actually respond. The response is the same for all three diseases: *Sanctify yourself!*

> *Now may the God of peace Himself sanctify you entirely; and may your spirit and soul and body be preserved complete, without blame at the coming of our Lord Jesus Christ.*
>
> 1 Thessalonians 5:23 NASB

There are a number of reasons, then, for disease. If you want easy, simple, step 1-2-3 answers, you won't find them here. You may ask, "Can the cause of my disease be determined?" That is the challenge facing the church today. The answer I can offer you is, *Yes!* I believe that some members of the body of Christ are especially equipped to help you. In an appropriate setting, if they know you and your private world, then through the work of the Holy Spirit they could give you a reasonably good idea why you or your loved one has a disease.

Will knowing the reason for a disease heal you? For some people it will, and for others it won't. I can't give you a definitive answer, because everyone is unique and circumstances are complex. However, I do know that the Lord cares greatly about your health and that your personal relationship with Him can change your health, depending on how you respond to Him. I am an ordinary man, and I will never heal anyone. Healing is the work of the Holy Spirit upon the directive of God the Father. But I can tell you that knowing the spiritual root cause will only help you. It will make you a more mature believer, and you will walk in closer fellowship with the Lord.

Having read the list of reasons for sickness, you might be wondering why my wife died. Let me give you my personal testimony.

On December 23, 2001, three months after diagnosis, we were out of town at Christmastime visiting Teresa's parents. Teresa had recently received a chemotherapy treatment and was experiencing nausea, so late that evening she was ill and in the bathroom for a while. Her family realized that she needed to be alone, so they decided to leave and go to her sister's house. That left Teresa and me alone for the rest of the night. When she felt better, we slept in her parents' bed and were cozy and warm all night long. It was very pleasant.

At about 2:00 a.m., I woke up. I could tell by her breathing that Teresa was not asleep, so I whispered, "Are you awake?" She replied that she was, so we got to snuggle and talk for a while. Then I decided to pray for her. I sat up and put my hands on her and started to pray out loud all the promises that I had been memorizing from God's Word. Then I heard what I call an "interrupting thought" in my head. Others have called it an "inner voice." This thought was as clear as if our young son had been standing in the room and begun talking to me. I had never heard such a voice before, and Teresa did not hear it. I stopped praying in mid-sentence because the voice was so loud. It said, "Klay, I am calling Teresa home because it serves my purpose. I will take care of you." Then I heard it a second time, with no other thoughts in my mind. The message was undeniable.

Remember, I was the guy who didn't believe such things. I had never been taught that God could talk to us in this manner. I had heard other people's testimonies, but to be honest, I was always skeptical. Some Christians seem to go overboard on this subject and get a word from God that they should order tater-tots instead of French fries! Well, the first thing that came to mind was that I had heard the voice of a demon and that I should test the spirits (1 John 4:1). Then I decided to keep it to myself, because I didn't want anyone to put me into a straightjacket or make me go to therapy. It wasn't until the next summer, when Teresa was in excellent health, that I told her and a few family members about that night. Understandably, no one really knew what to say.

In the twenty-sixth month, after the cancer had recurred, I told a dear friend and pastor about that night, and he reminded me of John 15:14-15. In that verse, Jesus calls his disciples "friends" and tells them that while slaves do not know what their master is doing, Jesus, as a friend, has told them what the Father is doing. My pastor said that it was possible the Lord was telling me these things as my friend. Yet I did not want to receive that message. It couldn't be true. I was still hoping that I would not have to live without my dear wife and best friend. But I understood what my pastor was saying. I was not completely convinced, however, so I asked the Lord for one more confirmation.

A week or so later, Teresa and I were listening to the Bible on CD. We were listening to John 10, which describes how the sheep of the town are put into the same pen for the night. In the morning, the shepherd calls his sheep *by name*, and they follow him because they know his voice (v. 3). Then the light came on in my mind, and I understood. My favorite seminary professor, Dr. Norman Geisler, said in one of his lectures to "look for the handprint of God." I know now that it was the voice of the Lord that night in 2001, because God called Teresa and me *by name*. It was his handprint. He was being kind to me and comforting me.

Many people have said to me, "I don't know how you get through this." Well, the way I make sense of it is that the Lord called Teresa home because *it served His purpose*. To the Lord, death is not punishment. It served His purpose that Teresa live through the disease and go home on that day according to His perfect plan. I don't fully understand His purpose, and I'm sure I will not fully understand until I stand in His presence. But at least I have the comfort of knowing that it wasn't a random tragedy or needless and wasteful loss of life. Don't misunderstand me; Teresa and I have had many sin issues in our lives (and I will be quick to admit that they were mostly mine). But I could not find a connection between a sin issue and the disease that she dealt with. I take it by faith that it all serves His purpose.

Now let's look more closely at the explanations given in Scripture for sickness. Here are the Bible references and rationale behind the seven reasons, along with some helpful illustrations.

1. *God's wrath*

   In Exodus, God used disease as a tool to make His point with the Egyptians (Exodus 15:26). In Isaiah, God sent a wasting disease among the stout warriors of Assyria (Isaiah 10:16). In Chronicles 21:14-15, Jehoram, king of Judah, fell from the favor of the Lord, and as a consequence experienced a severe sickness in his bowels. And in 1 Samuel 5 and 6, the Lord poured out his wrath upon the Philistines because they had taken the Ark of God. They were smitten with tumors until they returned the Ark to the Israelites at Ekron.

In each situation, there were unique circumstances. Groups of people were affected by disease, and each situation involved political and spiritual issues.

I would never put limits on the sovereign Creator of the universe, yet I do not consider this reason for disease as God's primary *modus operandi* in this day and age. It's certainly possible, but less likely, that the Lord would act in this manner with an individual saint in the church age, because we are living in a time after the cross and a time that is covered by grace. There are other reasons that are more rational and scripturally based, so I will not linger on this first reason.

2. *Sins of others*

In 2 Samuel 24:1-17, we read the familiar story of how King David became proud of the strength of Israel and commanded Joab, his military commander, to go and number all the fighting men. David's loyal advisors told him not to do it, but he refused their advice. As a consequence, David was disciplined by God and, through the prophet Gad, even given the opportunity to choose his punishment. David chose three days of pestilence or plague. He says plainly in verse 17, "I have sinned and I have done wrong." He asked the Lord to put the punishment upon Him and his house and not upon the innocent sheep of Israel. Nevertheless, in those three days, over 70,000 men of Israel died because of David's sin. Scriptures do not mention the number of women and children who died, but I am certain the number was significant.

Additional examples show how the sin of one man affected others, although not necessarily resulting in disease. In the case of Korah's rebellion in Numbers 16, all of his wives and their families—children, grandchildren and all—were swallowed up by the earth and killed. It just doesn't seem fair! If I were there, I'd say, "Hey Grandpa, I'm going to stand over here to the side for a moment until this meeting is over, okay?" Nevertheless, it's true. We do not live on a desert island, for sin affects others. In the case of the sin of Achan in Joshua 7, thirty-six soldiers were killed in battle. Their death left an undetermined number of widows and orphans in the camp, and in turn changed their lives and the lives of their descendants. All of it happened because of the sin of one man.

I remember a modern-day story of a woman who contracted HIV. She acquired the virus through her husband. She was a faithful woman, but her husband was not a faithful man. He had acquired the virus through sexually promiscuous behavior in a second life that he conducted in secret outside their marriage. In the end, they both died, and their child was orphaned and raised by family members. Did the woman have the disease because of anything she did? No. Did those who died in Israel due to the plague brought on by King David's sin do anything wrong? No. They had a disease caused by the sin of others.

3. *Sins of our ancestral fathers*

God "will by no means leave the guilty unpunished, visiting the iniquity of the fathers on the children and on the grandchildren to the third and fourth generations" (Ex 34:7 NASB). This is repeated in Exodus 20:5 in the context of the Ten Commandments. I realize that this took place during a time in history when the people were required to live by the Levitical law, and some will argue that this no longer applies because the law has passed away. However, the law is not the focus when we consider this passage for this application. The law reflects the character of God. It is *His character* that must be considered in this passage. Although we may not fully understand it, one of the characteristics of sin is that it has generational consequences.

So what about the infant born with a genetic disease? What did he do to deserve such a difficult life? What about the other hundreds of thousands of people who are genetically predisposed to certain diseases, such as diabetes? I met one lady who had brain cancer at age thirty-six. When she was a child, her father had died of the exact same disease, at age thirty-six. Did any of these people do something personally to deserve the health issues they're dealing with? No, probably not. However, they bear responsibility regarding their *response* to the disease, although not in the acquisition of it.

Have you ever noticed how certain behavior patterns follow families? Some of the behavior is admirable, and some of it is shameful. Abraham was caught lying in Genesis 20:2 when he told Abimelech, King of Gerar, that Sarah was his sister. Technically speaking, she was his half-sister, but he hid the critical fact that she was also his wife. Isaac also lied in Genesis 26:7 when the men of Gerar asked about Rebecca. Isaac feared the men and told them Rebecca was his sister. Jacob lied to Isaac in Genesis 27:24 when he told him that he was Esau. Jacob stole Esau's blessing as a result. Then, in Genesis chapter 37, we read of the conflict between the sons of Jacob. It all culminates in the lie told to Jacob that a wild beast had killed Joseph. Four generations recorded in the Scriptures, and four generations of lying behavior.

Generational patterns can be found in many areas of our lives and can be both good and bad. They can be disease-related through genetics, or emotional or social, or even matters of lifestyle. I know of one family with three generations of pastors, and I've read of another family with five medical doctors. There are many examples of this. I have knowledge of one family in which the grandfather was emotionally and sexually abusive to his wife and family. His daughter left home at age sixteen and was married only a few months later. Because of her abusive home life, she was poorly equipped to parent. As a result, her children were poorly equipped to deal with the social pressures, and one of her daughters became pregnant out of wedlock at age seventeen. She delivered the child amid feelings of shame and guilt. That child was born premature and had a stroke at birth. She is now living her life moderately handicapped.

I recognize that each individual makes choices and can break these patterns if they desire to do so. However, I still ask, what if that original home, the home of the grandfather, had been a God-fearing home? What if it had been a home of security, warmth, and peace? Could things have been different? Is it possible that the fruit of their behavior worked its way down the family tree and eventually led to a child who now lives with a handicap? I think it's possible, although there is no way to know for certain. I believe that godly behavior would have led to blessings. I believe that the daughter, granddaughter, and great-granddaughter would have been more likely to live peaceful and fulfilling lives if the grandfather had provided Christian leadership. But this did not happen. It is my belief that the iniquity of the father was visited upon the children and on the grandchildren to the third and fourth generations.

I want to add that there is a scriptural example of a proper response to the sins of the fathers. In Nehemiah 1:6 and 9:2, the people of Israel acknowledged the sins of their fathers and asked for forgiveness. In Daniel 9:15-19, the prophet Daniel also acknowledged the sins of his fathers and asked that he be forgiven of those sins. In Psalms 106, the Psalter acknowledged the sins of his generational fathers in his discourse of praise to God.

Each person is held accountable for his or her own sin. I cannot ask forgiveness for something my grandfather did. He must ask for forgiveness himself. I can, however, acknowledge that there was sin and that it has affected me. I can pray and renounce that sin and ask God to remove the consequences of that sin *in my life and for the generations to come.* That prayer can break the curses that seem to follow families. It serves as a clear statement of faith and intent to serve the "one, true, living God." Through this prayer we can declare our intentions to renounce the work of Satan in our lives, akin to Joshua's statement, "As for me and my house, we shall serve the Lord" (Joshua 24:15).

4. *Our own sin*

There is a television commercial airing today for a weight loss pill. The advertising script is memorable: "Have you gained weight? Well, it's not your fault!" This reminds me of the events in the Garden of Eden (Gen 3:12-13). When confronted with his act of disobedience, Adam was quick to blame it on his wife. "It was Eve's fault!" he said. When Eve was confronted, she just as quickly blamed the serpent. It's the same today. *People are very reluctant to admit their own sin.* As the commercial says, "It's not my fault." But the truth is, we do sin, and we are the cause of many of our own diseases because of the way we live. We must take responsibility for our actions and for what we put into our minds.

Psalm 38 is a sorrowful chapter. King David was suffering with a disease that caused burning in his loins. He says plainly in verse 3: "There is no health in my bones because of my sin." Yes, we have security in our eternal salvation, and our sins are forgiven. However, *there are still consequences to many sins in this life.* There is no avoiding it. Yes, the power of sin has been removed; sin cannot separate us from a relationship with our heavenly Father. But again, there are still consequences for sin. We cannot keep on sinning so that grace may abound (Rom 6:1-2). There is also an eternal consequence to sin with respect to rewards in heaven. Unfortunately, most people want to be like Adam and Eve, or even like the saleswoman with the weight loss pill, and say, "It's not my fault!" Well, that's simply not true. I'd like to tell you otherwise, but I would be lying. The passages in Exodus 15:26 and Deuteronomy 28, when considered from the perspective that they reflect the character of God, also teach as a general principle that sin has consequences and that there is a reward for obedience. I will expand on the workings of this process in the following chapters.

I want to repeat: people don't like to admit to their sin because of pride or because of the pain it will cause. I am concerned that readers will jump to my next reason, the purpose of God, as an explanation for their disease because they refuse to examine or take responsibility for sin in their own lives. In my opinion, in most situations the person who is affected by the disease cannot draw an objective conclusion about themselves. Typically, they are blinded to the error of their ways. I believe that an elder or pastor in the church who has been given the opportunity to talk with the person and know his or her private thoughts is the best person to evaluate the situation. (I will discuss this further in chapter seven.) If the elder is unable to draw a conclusion, then look to another person. Godly spouses, parents, and children are in excellent positions to discern the matters of the affected person's private world. I can think of one man who was bound by anxiety so badly that he couldn't hold a job. But if you asked him, he would say he was "just fine" and that his situation "served the purpose of God." If the truth were told, he was in denial and did not want to take responsibility for his actions.

In 1 Corinthians 11:26-32, we read that God does, in fact, discipline us as saints when we do not examine our lives or repent of our sin even when we take communion.

> *For as often as you eat this bread and drink the cup, you proclaim the Lord's death until He*

> *comes. Therefore, whoever eats the bread or drinks the cup of the Lord in an unworthy manner, shall be guilty of the body and the blood of the Lord. But a man must examine himself, and in so doing he is to eat of the bread and drink of the cup. For he who eats and drinks, eats and drinks judgment to himself if he does not judge the body rightly. For this reason many among you are weak and sick, and a number sleep. But if we judged ourselves rightly, we would not be judged. But when we are judged, we are disciplined by the Lord so that we will not be condemned along with the world. (NASB)*

God is capable of disciplining us even outside the context of sin, as discussed in Hebrews 12:5-11. How much more will we be disciplined if we sin? Will we become like the ungodly in Romans 1:24 who, even though they knew God, did not honor him or give thanks? God gave them over to the lusts of their hearts, to impurity and more. How much more will He deal with His beloved saints when they allow sin to control areas of their lives?

James 5:16 also deals with sin and sickness: "Therefore confess your sins to one another, and pray for one another so that you may be healed." There is great disagreement over the word *healed* in the passage. The root word in Greek is *iaomai* (#2390 in *Strong's Concordance*). The first definition of the word is "physical healing," with a supplemental meaning, "to be made whole." I don't see much conflict between those words. One is good, and the other is even better. They both lead to healing and identify sin as the root cause. The second definition is "figurative language of spiritual healing," but as you will see, spiritual wholeness almost always relates directly to physical healing.

I will not suggest to you that I have the scriptural insight to resolve the debate that has existed for decades. I can tell you—and you will better understand this after reading the next chapter—that our bodies have the miraculous ability to heal on their own. Healing is part of God's perfect design. So if a sin issue is the cause of the disease, and that sin issue is removed through confession and changed behavior, then the body has an opportunity to heal. There are other situations in which the body is so badly damaged that it would require a creative miracle from the Lord to restore health. In other cases, the disease may remain but no longer progresses. I have heard credible testimony of all of these events occurring. Healing is a gift from God, and His ways are not our ways. "As far as the heavens are above the earth are His ways above our ways and His thoughts above our thoughts" (Isaiah 55:8-9). So I cannot explain why some people are healed and some people are not. I can safely say, however, that we are far better off when we set aside pride and admit that we have sinned.

The most obvious example of disease brought on by our own sin would be those connected with sexual promiscuity. Sexually transmitted diseases are everywhere. God has designed sex for one man and one woman within the context of marriage. Sexual sin also carries with it consequences that are social, emotional, and spiritual. I can quickly think of four men who left the ministry as a consequence of problems in this area.

As you continue reading, you will see the complete picture of how sin can cause disease.

5. *The Lord's purpose*

In John 9, we read the story of the man who was blind since birth. The disciples asked Jesus, "Who sinned, this man or his parents?" (The disciples were familiar with reasons #3 and #4 above.) Jesus responded that it was neither; the man was born blind so that the works of God would be displayed in him. His healing caused a great uproar in the local synagogue. The Pharisees were infuriated that the man had been healed. In addition to the purpose that it fulfilled at that moment, a full chapter of John was devoted to the event and included in God's Word for our benefit for all time.

The suffering of Job is also an example of God's purpose. When I read the story of Job, I think, "Hey God, whose side are you on? Why did you mention his name to Satan?" If He hadn't mentioned Job's name, Job could have avoided all that suffering. What we need to understand is that, when God allows this kind of thing to happen, His goals are not usually our goals. God is not impressed with the house we live in or the money we've made or the diplomas we have. All those things get left here when we die. His values are spiritual in nature, values such as the fruit of the spirit: love, joy, peace, patience, kindness, goodness, faithfulness, and self-control. Is it possible that He wanted to build these values into the life of Job? He desires that we keep our eyes on Him.

I can also tell you that God's timetable is not our timetable. For me, patience means that I wait a good long thirty minutes. Then I observe my daughter, who has cerebral palsy, and how she waits for hours for friends to call or rides to arrive. I know that her circumstances will last her entire lifetime. There's a big difference between what I call patience and what she calls patience. It's the same with the Lord. Sometimes He's trying to get through to us. Who has the right to question the sovereign God of all creation? Our proper response is to have faith in Him and His Word.

Finally, Paul writes that when we are weak, our Lord is strong (2 Cor 12:10). What this means is that, when we no longer rely on our own abilities and trust in the Lord's ability, then we are accomplishing the purpose that God intended.

I have spent hours trying to understand God's purpose for intervening in my life and calling home my dear wife at age thirty-eight. Will this disease change my children or our families in some way that God desires? Will it change me? Will there possibly be a change in the life of someone whom Teresa knew? Perhaps there will be a change in the life of someone whom God will bring into my life, or perhaps a generational purpose. I have found comfort in Isaiah 57:1, which states that the righteous are taken away to protect them from the evil to come. Yes, the Lord might have been protecting Teresa from something in the future. Simply stated, I do not know the purpose of God. I simply walk in faith that God is sovereign, that He loves me and Teresa, and that this is what He ordained. God is all good all the time. He is perfect and loving in all his ways. Praise God for who He is!

6. *God is calling us home*

2 Kings 13:14 begins: "When Elisha became sick with the illness of which he was to die . . ." Because of the fall of man, Adam's sin in the Garden of Eden, every man must die. There is no escaping it. We will all die. Some of us will die in accidents. Some will die quickly from such things as heart attacks or strokes. Others will die of disease. When Elisha was called home, God allowed a disease to be the cause of the end of his life.

Most of us hope that when it's our time to go home, we go home quickly. However, I think that there are times when the disease process is actually a time to allow everyone involved an opportunity to prepare for separation. I've heard it said that it's common for the person who is sick to help and bless the caregivers more than the caregivers help and bless the one who is sick. I think this was true in my case. Teresa prepared me for my life without her.

Nevertheless, this is a biblical reason for disease. God is calling us home. I pray that the Lord will be gracious and merciful to my family and me when that day arrives.

7. *Any combination of the above*

    In Numbers 12, we have the story of Moses' sister Miriam, who, with her brother Aaron, sinned against the Lord. They spoke against Moses because he married a Cushite woman. The Lord's anger burned against them, and Miriam became leprous. Moses, the most humble of all men (Num 12:3), pleaded before God to remove the disease. The Lord heard the prayer of Moses, but He also required Miriam to be separated from the camp for seven days. Miriam's disease was brought on by her own sin, but God used the situation to fulfill His purpose when He restored her after the required seven days. This serves as an example of God's wrath, the consequences of our own sin, and God's purpose, all in one passage. This is important to note, because it can still occur today. Someone may have a disease for multiple reasons.

    This concludes the seven reasons for diseases found in the Scriptures. Next I will discuss how Satan can steal our health, a three-step process involving three seemingly unrelated subjects.

Chapter 2

Puzzle Piece #1 of 3: A Closer Look at Sin

Remember the old boast, "I don't cuss, smoke, or chew, and I don't go with girls who do!" Most of the illustrations of sin that I remember hearing in sermons over the years have been of sins against the flesh, such as cussing, smoking, and chewing. Sexual sins get a lot of attention, along with dealing drugs and drunk driving. These are followed closely by satanic rituals and gang activity. Well, since I don't participate in any of those things, I guess I'm pearly white and 99.99% sinless, right?

Actually, the above statement couldn't be further from the truth. My point is that I don't understand why the more common sins are not mentioned as often. In this chapter, I want to broaden the definition of sin to include the invisible sins. I believe that most of the sins that reside unopposed in the lives of the saints are the *sins against the spirit*, rather than those against the flesh. In the following chapter, I will discuss four very common sins. However, this list is not complete. In fact, sins against the spirit make a long list.

The first and most prevalent sin against the spirit is fear. Fear, which also goes by the name of *worry* or *anxiety*, can manifest in many forms: fear of losing one's job, fear of financial failure, fear of the death of a child or other loved one, fear of people, fear of confrontation, or fear of taking responsibility for our own actions. There is fear of social rejection, fear of commitment, fear of sexual infidelity of our spouse, and even fear caused by performance-based love, to name a few. This list can include the smallest of issues.

Second, yet still at the top of the list of sins against the spirit, is bitterness, or unforgiveness. Other sins against the spirit include guilt, self-hatred and self-rejection, envy, conditional love (performance-based), self-pity, lack of joy in our heavenly Father, occult involvement (even unintentional), intellectual idolatry and pride, and accusation. Accusation can be understood as criticism or judgment that is inappropriate, first seen in Satan in Genesis 3:4 in his dialogue with Eve. The list goes on and on. Sins against the spirit that are invisible are still sin, even if they are not sins of the flesh!

One reasonable definition of sin is "any deviation from the perfect character of God." Part of our life journey as Christians is to be molded into His image. This is sanctification. If we're honest, most of us will admit to some sin in our lives. But the most difficult sin to identify and turn away from is the sin that we are not aware of, sin that has built itself into our character so deep that it becomes part of us. That was the case in my life. One of my biggest sin issues was simply part of my personality. Experts teach that the most difficult step in the process of alcohol or drug rehabilitation is acknowledging that you have a problem. Well, that was me! As far as I was concerned, I didn't have a sin issue. The truth was that you couldn't separate me from my sin; I was in partnership with it. It wasn't until my spiritual eyes were opened and I began to see the character of God that I finally recognized my sin. On that day, I confessed my sin and renounced my behavior and have not returned to it since.

> *The most difficult sin to identify and turn away from is the sin that we are not aware of. It is sin that has built itself into our character so deep that it becomes us!*

Fear

Let me give you an example of fear in my life. When my wife was first diagnosed, my response was one of sin, not faith. I fell victim to a deep-seated fear. For the next three months, I held a daily pity party in my private world. It was a big party, and I invited everyone that my imagination could hold. I went so far that I even planned my wife's prospective funeral in every detail, and she wasn't even near death! I had the location picked out, the music, the speakers, and all the special testimonies. Of course, I did all of this in the privacy of my own mind. There was no one around to point out my behavior. And I must be honest . . . Even if someone had offered me help, I don't think I would have listened, at least not until the day I was told that fear was a sin. What? Fear, a sin? *No, no, no*, I thought. *Fear is a natural human emotion.*

Of course, in the case of an immediate threat to safety, fear is justified, such as when you need to get out of the way of that sixteen-year-old boy speeding down the street in his new sports car. Then, fear is acceptable. But the *sustained* fear that is imbedded in one's personality and causes lifestyle and behavior changes is sin. Sinful fear is fear that becomes part of our thought process and influences our decisions, and which prompts unexplained and compulsive action. Yes, all of this is in conflict with God's Word. There are hundreds of times in the Scriptures when we are commanded, "Do not be afraid," or "Fear not," or "Do not fear" (1 John 4:18, John 14:27, Rom 8:15 NASB, and 2 Tim 1:7, translated *fear* in KJV). Fear is the opposite of faith. With faith comes peace, and peace is part of the kingdom of God (Rom 14:17). "And without faith it is impossible to please Him" (Heb 11:6).

I have seen women live in constant fear at home. They fear that their husbands will not like the food they prepare. One woman feared that her husband would become upset if she got home late or if she refused his romantic overtures. Sometimes the fear comes only from within the woman's thought life, and sometimes it comes from the husband. Sometimes it's a combination. In my own marriage, I had to learn that I could incite fear without even knowing it. Therefore, my wife and I both brought about changes in our behavior to put us more in line with the way God wanted us to live.

Domestic abuse is widespread in the church, both emotional and physical, and it affects all age groups and all social classes. Sometimes a spouse is physically present but emotionally absent. This abandonment is common and can lead to fear, eventually stealing an individual's health.

Let me give an example of fear as a sin by contrasting two students. One lives with fear in his life, while the other does not. On the same day, they both decide to enroll in the local community college. Within a week, the healthy student has gone to the campus, submitted an application, and registered for classes; he's ready for the next semester. The fearful student, however, has not fared so well. Because of fear, he's reluctant even to go to campus. What is he afraid of? Perhaps he's afraid of the unknown, or perhaps failure or risk. So he puts it off until the very last day. When he pulls into the parking lot, he drives around for a long time because he doesn't know which building to go to and is afraid that the campus security guard is watching him and will give him a ticket if he parks in the wrong place. Finally he parks and, with eyes on the ground, walks onto campus. Because he's still lost, he's afraid people are looking at him and will consider him stupid, so he doesn't make eye contact with anyone. Instead, he pretends he's waiting on a friend as he lingers around the buildings. Finally he comes across a campus map and finds a building marked *Student Center*, so he decides to go there. Once inside, he follows signs for new students, but he struggles with each step: the application process, the registration process, the bookstore, everything. By the end of the afternoon, he's exhausted. He has only enrolled in three of the five classes, because the other two classes he wanted were filled on the last day.

Do you relate to any part of this illustration? Do you know someone like this? Do you see how fear can make it into our thought processes and actually *become* our thinking? Do you know people who are anxious and frequently worried? Is this how the Lord wants us to live? We have all allowed fear into our lives on some level.

I have seen employers motivate their employees through intimidation. I have been threatened with the loss of my job, and, until I recognized it, I worked in a constant state of fear. I have been present during shouting matches and near fistfights in the secular workplace. All of this comes out of fear. As a Christian man, I was already honoring the Lord and putting forth my best effort. Using fear as a motivational tactic was most ineffective and destructive at that company. Fear is not a part of the Kingdom of God or what God has for you, one of his beloved. It will only produce stress in your body and increase your exposure to disease.

In time, God took care of my family and me. He had something much better in mind for us. So do not fear!

Now I ask, can God bless me if my thoughts are bound up in fear? Will God bless me if I verbalize fear? Can He bless me if I am in partnership with a sin such as fear in an area of my life? When I act in fear and not faith, I am actually giving glory to and being obedient to the kingdom of darkness. What happens to the presence of the Holy Spirit in our lives when we speak words of fear? How long can we allow sin to be present in our lives and not expect to face its consequences? Can we expect to receive God's blessing and protection when we continue to partner with sin in a certain area of our life? This is a difficult question, but the answer is clear: No, we cannot. God will eventually discipline us.

I believe that our heavenly Father makes the decision regarding when to allow the consequences of sin. There is no way to predict when you are about to face consequences. In the case of Job, the timing of his suffering seemed so arbitrary. Prior to the events recorded in Job 1, there was a hedge of protection around him. In an instant, it was lifted. There was no step 1-2-3 process provided in the Scriptures that would explain to us why God did what He did. Perhaps this trial was a result of the fear that resided in Job's life (as expressed in v. 3:25)

How long do you think you can allow sin to be present in your life before you face the consequences? What if it's a sin that you have not recognized or acknowledged? How long can you establish Satan's kingdom in an area of your life before it manifests itself in some way?

Accusation

I wonder how many times on any given Sunday at the local church, a woman thinks, *I wish I had hair as pretty as the lady sitting in front of me.* Or maybe it's the other way around: *That lady's hair looks awful! She looks downright stupid.* Or perhaps, *She should not be singing a solo this morning; I'm a much better singer than she is. They just don't appreciate me.* These are all thoughts based on accusation, in which we pass judgment, compare ourselves to another, and demonstrate envy. They are all sins against our spirit.

This sin is first seen in Genesis 3:1 in Satan's dialogue with the Eve. First the serpent asked, "You shall not eat from any tree of the garden," which he knew was not what God had commanded. Then he said in verse 4, "You will not die." In short, he accused God of wrongdoing. Satan had removed himself from being under the authority of God, and he wanted to do it his own way.

In the church, we all matter. We all have roles to play, from childcare to property maintenance. There is no role that is more important than another. We must put ourselves under the authority of God and find that place where he leads us to serve. This is a drastically different attitude from one of accusation.

Lack of Joy in the Father

In my own life, I have been guilty of the sin of having a lack of joy. I have let the worries of the world grow so large that they have taken the joy of my Father from me. Have you ever been asked by a friend, "What has taken your joy?" This is a great question! In my case, it was any number of issues. That is my point. There was *always something* to keep me from saying, "Thank you, Father," and having that "attitude of gratitude." Joy is a character trait of our heavenly Father, and lack of joy in Him is a sin against our spirit. It's not a *suggestion,* it's a *command* that we should be joyful in the Lord always (Phil 4:4). *Joy, overjoyed, enjoy, rejoice* . . . The terms we find in the Scriptures all refer to the same attitude. Remember the times when you've met old friends and talked about the good old days? You tell stories and relive the past; you laugh and have a good time. Well, rejoicing in the Lord is like that, too. Take pleasure in what He has done in your life. Relive the "good old days" when you experienced His love and kindness in your life.

I wonder what our Heavenly Father thinks when we gather 80,000 people in a stadium. We bring a marching band and some pretty cheerleaders, dress in the same colors, and then yell at the top of our lungs when our favorite team scores a touchdown. The marching band plays until they are exhausted, and then everyone goes home to read the newspaper and Internet news the next day. We talk about the victory for a week. But in some churches, when someone professes their faith for the first time or is baptized, we sit stoically and respond with polite applause. Shouldn't these two responses actually be reversed? Shouldn't we celebrate when someone receives salvation? Shouldn't we show a little more joy in the Father? What is really important?

I've also found it interesting that some of the most joyful people I've ever known are those with the fewest material possessions, so I know that joy is not tied to having more "stuff." I've learned that having joy in my heavenly Father is a matter of the heart and not based on the material possessions around me.

Bitterness

I am also the king of bitterness. Next to fear, bitterness is perhaps the second most destructive sin against the spirit. Let me give you another word of testimony. In May of 1988, six weeks prior to my marriage with Teresa, she and I were falsely accused by our state's child protection agency of sexually abusing her two children (the children I later adopted). I believe that this was Satan's attempt to destroy our future family. I won't give the details, because that would be a whole book in itself. I will simply tell you that none of the accusations were true, and the state had no case. Even their own expert testified against the state's child protection workers. The matter should have been resolved within a few days. However, that agency continued to press the issue in court. With the Lord's blessing of two excellent attorneys, we countersued the state. Four and a half years later, we won a precedent-setting case in the Texas Supreme Court when the case was deemed frivolous. We won reimbursement of our attorney's fees, which had accumulated to over $70,000. For me personally, however, it wasn't over for another fifteen years.

There were three people who were primarily responsible for the actions of the state. As it turned out, one of them—I'll call him Joe—lived in my suburb less than three miles from my house. A few years later, he ran for an elected office in my city. My bitterness toward him remained, and I did everything I could to prevent him from being elected and re-elected for several years running. I can't tell you how many hours I spent stewing in my anger toward Joe and his two colleagues. I was confident that he deserved every insult I could direct his way.

Then one day at a church conference, a dear Christian man eighty years old spoke to me of my bitterness. Amazingly, I did not see myself as bitter. Instead, I rationalized that I was a victim and that I was entitled to get even. Yet how could I argue with this kind, elderly saint? He told me that I must release Joe to the Lord. I must forgive him, or I would not be forgiven. He told me that Joe, just like myself, made mistakes, and that Joe's life and his sanctification were not my responsibility, but the Lord's. He reminded me of Jesus' statements on the cross: "Lord, forgive them, for they know not what they are doing" (Luke 23:34). I didn't fully understand the consequences of my own actions. I had embraced and rationalized bitterness until it *was me*. I had a partner named Bitterness, and he was such a close buddy that you couldn't see light between us. Sin had

> *I had rationalized bitterness and embraced bitterness until it was me. You couldn't see light between us!*

become manifest in me, and I am fortunate that I do not have a disease today because of my bitterness.

Other Sins of the Spirit

Here is a complex question about spiritual sins: Are we responsible for sin that we are not aware of? These are also sins against our spirit. I'm talking about sin that has made its way into our character, such as vanity, low self-esteem, suspicion, and guilt. Is an alcoholic still responsible for his behavior even if he doesn't recognize that he's an alcoholic? The answer is yes. We are responsible for the sins that we have committed in ignorance. There are consequences for those sins, too. This is made clear in the Old Testament. Under the Levitical law, the priest made sacrifices for sins committed in ignorance (Ez 45:19-20 and Heb 9:7).

I'll provide an example of a sin committed in ignorance. I believe that God desires that we take all things to him in prayer (Eph 6:18, Phil 4:6, 1 Thess 5:16) and I also believe that taking medicine without prayer is wrong. It's not so much the fact that we take the medicine, but the attitude that we demonstrate when we take the medicine without prayer. I realize that this topic is controversial. Therefore, let me defend my claim.

> *For many of us, prescription drugs are only a symptomatic treatment that actually prevents us from addressing the root problem, which is actually spiritual.*

Today, prescription drugs are big business and part of everyday life in America. One recent CNN article stated that 40% of the American population is on some type of medication. There are those who need their medication so badly that they can't live without it. I recognize that for some, such as diabetics, the medication is lifesaving. But for many others, medication is only a symptomatic treatment that actually prevents them from addressing the true root problem, which is actually a spiritual matter, either in part or in whole. To make matters worse, one medication often leads to another, and then another. The first medication might have a side effect that makes you nauseated and keeps you from sleeping. So you add two more medicines, an anti-nausea medication and something to help you sleep. It goes on and on from there, until you're taking pills all day. As I said previously, doctors don't pastor, so they are often limited to just one treatment for you, and that is to write a prescription. I don't believe that God wants this for you. Let me explain further with a word of testimony.

About six months after Teresa died, two close friends told me that they thought I met the clinical definition for depression and that I should go to the doctor to get an antidepressant. They were well intended, and yes, I was depressed for a legitimate reason; I was grieving the loss of my loved one. However, I'm not too keen on putting chemicals in my body, especially those that alter my mind. So with prayerful thought, I sought another answer. What would God have me do? I asked him for wisdom and for his perfect solution.

As a result, I found two options. First, I decided that it would be wiser to start an exercise program primarily centered on jogging. I have a wonderful park near my home with a three-mile loop trail, so I went out and walked it five days a week for about two weeks. Then I began to walk and run the trail, and each time, I tried to run farther. Well, that went on for about eight weeks, until I was able to actually run the entire distance slowly, without stopping. I felt wonderful that day because I had achieved something. I increased the program from there. Eventually, after about six months, I extended my distance to five miles and began tracking my times to see if I could run faster. I was still grieving, but I had a better way of addressing the problem. I believe that it was what the Lord preferred for me over a medication that provided chemical stimulation. After a good run, I felt good, no doubt about it. I lost weight, and my body became toned. I've always heard that exercise helps us deal with stress, and I found it to be true.

It reduced my depression significantly. I'm certain that my body released the "feel-good endorphins" as a result of my physical activity.

The second solution the Lord showed me was to sing, so I joined the choir at my church. Do you know how difficult it is to be depressed and sing praises to God at the same time? It's almost impossible! I bought my choir's CD and an album of the old traditional hymns that I used to sing while sitting next to my grandmother at church. What great memories, and what great songs! For me, the depression leaves whenever I sing "Christ the Lord Is Risen Today," "Holy, Holy, Holy," and "O For a Thousand Tongues to Sing," to name a few. I challenge you to sing uplifting songs of praise when you're depressed. The songs will take your mind off of yourself and take away the sinful thoughts of self-pity that often accompany depression, and put them on your Heavenly Father. God inhabits praise! Do you want to hear some great news? The biblical truths of God do not change with our emotions. Our emotions come and go like the blowing of the wind, but biblical truths are as rock-solid as granite.

> *Biblical truths do not change with our emotions. They are as rock-solid as granite.*

On the other hand, I will tell you that Teresa and I did pray over the treatments and medication she received. She made her own decisions, accepting some and rejecting others. I am not opposed to medical treatments; I know the Lord can use a doctor to heal just as easily as not. The Lord used the doctors' treatments to extend Teresa's life an additional two years. The decision to take medicine is a personal decision. My best recommendation is to make it a matter of prayer. Make a slow decision with prayer.

I'm reminded of King Nebuchadnezzar in Daniel 1:20, and I feel that I was in a similar situation. In every matter of wisdom and understanding about which the king consulted Daniel, Hananiah, Mishael, and Azariah, he found the wisdom of God to be ten times better than all the magicians and conjurers in all his realm. So I ask you, do you rely on the wisdom of God regarding your health treatments? Do you pray about them?

Continuing with the idea of unintentional sin, some will argue that today's drugs are a modern-day form of witchcraft and sorcery, and that taking medication could possibly open your life to satanic involvement. The basis of this argument surrounds the usage of the Greek word *pharmakeia* (*Strong's* #5331) and its place in Galatians 5:20. *Pharmakeia* is the root word of our English word *pharmacy*, which means, "the art and place of making and dispensing medicine." I think both sides in this argument raise legitimate issues. In the pre-modern era, there was not much of a difference between medicine and sorcery. Tribal priests would concoct potions or "medicine" and use sorcery, which included incantations and spells, as they applied their treatments. This is clearly an invitation for satanic involvement in someone's life. In our modern era, however, medicine is typically scientifically based, and it must clear FDA approval and be prescribed by a licensed medical doctor or nurse practitioner before being used in this country.

Just because these medicines are scientifically based, however, does not mean that we no longer need God's involvement in our lives. Does science replace God? No, of course not. Even if a medication is scientifically proven, it will not necessarily be effective without God's blessing. God is sovereign over the most proven scientifically based medical treatments.

The world of alternative medicine is different from the allopathic establishment, and treatments can also become sins committed in ignorance. With alternative medicines, there may or may not be a scientific basis for the treatments. There is a long list of these treatments, which include acupuncture/acupressure, aromatherapy, hypnotherapy, iridology, magnetic healing, reflexology, and visualization, to name only a few. Some of these treatment methods have evolved from or incorporate parts of eastern religions and pantheism. A thousand questions come up when considering these therapies. What does the Lord think about them? Does He need them to bring healing to my body? Do they bring Him honor? Do they actually benefit me, and will they heal my disease?[1] This leads you to yet another personal decision and my conclusion on this subject: It is of the utmost importance that you seek the Lord before receiving any treatments for a disease.

Why is seeking the Lord so important to me? One of my favorite Old Testament stories is found in Numbers 21:4-9 (NASB):

> *Then they set out from Mount Hor by the way of the Red Sea, to go around the land of Edom; and the people became impatient because of the journey. The people spoke against God and Moses, "Why have you brought us up out of Egypt to die in the wilderness? For there is no food and no water, and we loathe this miserable food."*
>
> *The Lord sent fiery serpents among the people which bit the people, so that many people of Israel died. So the people came to Moses and said, "We have sinned, because we have spoken against the Lord and you; intercede with the Lord, that He may remove the serpents from us." And Moses interceded for the people. Then the Lord said to Moses, "Make a fiery serpent, and set it on a standard; and it shall come about, that everyone who is bitten, when he looks at it, he will live." And Moses made a*

[1] Probe Ministries has an informative article that is worth reading: "The Rise of Alternative Medicine," by Patrick Zukeran. It can be found at http://www.probe.org/content/view/16/0/.

> *bronze serpent and set it on the standard; and it came about, that if a serpent bit any man, when he looked to the bronze serpent, he lived.*

I think one of the lessons that we should learn from this passage is simply to look to the Lord—or at least to His provision for us, which was the bronze serpent in this passage—for our needs. We are commanded to pray without ceasing (1 Thess 5:17). The whole reason for Christ's death on the cross was so that we can have a personal relationship with our Father in heaven. So let's do it! Let's seek His wisdom, especially on the subject of medication.

Before I leave the subject of spiritual sins, I want to briefly touch on one additional subject that I consider critical to the subject of disease: our diet. Why would I discuss diet in the context of spiritual sins? It's because I believe that our culture-wide problem with eating is fundamentally a spiritual issue, one that manifests itself in a physical form. Allow me to elaborate on this subject.

The typical American diet is poor, and the average American is twenty pounds overweight. Reports vary, but as of 2005, one-third of adult Americans were considered obese. For the first time in history, the expected lifespan in our country has decreased because of this weight problem! It has become increasingly common for life insurance companies to decline overweight applicants.

One of the main consequences of overeating is diabetes. Adult-onset diabetes is at an all-time high level, and childhood diabetes has increased tenfold in the last twenty years. One recent report stated that sixty percent of all cancer deaths are preventable with regular exercise, better diet, and medical screenings. Of course, exercise, a healthy diet, and medical screenings are commonsense measures. There are numerous other studies that have proven that by reducing caloric intake and increasing the nutritional value of the food we eat, we can greatly reduce our risk of disease, increase our lifespan, and extend our vital years by up to forty percent (as documented in the excellent book *Beyond the 120 Year Diet*, by Roy Walford, M.D.).

So why do we overeat? Is it because we're hungry? Is there some genetic flaw from our ancestral fathers that makes us consume large quantities of food? No, in my observation, in a majority of the cases we eat for emotional satisfaction, or we eat with a spirit of gluttony. We eat to deal with stress. We desire to feel loved and significant, so we reach for comfort food, when in fact we should be opening our hearts to the Lord. Our comfort and our significance are found in Him, not in eating more food. Sometimes we eat in disregard for our body and the fact that it is the temple of the Holy Spirit. After seeking Him, we should naturally demonstrate one of the fruits of the spirit, self-control. That is a spiritual matter. Do you remember the television commercial I mentioned in Chapter 1, in which the lady says, "Have you gained weight? It's not your fault!" Well, most of the time it IS our fault—but we can change it with the help of the Holy Spirit.

I believe that fasting is very beneficial to the body and spirit and should be practiced today. Scriptures do not expressly command us to fast. However, Jesus taught us fasting by example (Matt 4:2) and he spoke of it as if it were a normal part of his life (Matt 6:16-18, Luke 8:15). It is my observation that most churches today ignore the subject and practice of fasting. I'm not sure why or when things changed. Apart from scriptural encouragement, there are many health benefits to fasting. In their excellent book *Prescription for Nutritional Healing*, James F. Balch, M.D., and Phyllis A Balch, CNC, recommend a three-day solid food fast once a month and a ten-day solid food fast twice a year (p. 548) just so the body can rest and detoxify. To understand correctly, realize that it is typically a solid food fast, not an absolute fast. A variety of nutritional fluids are recommended, as well as supervision and assistance from a health-care professional.

Now let me summarize puzzle piece #1 in the context of disease. I have clarified my working definition of sin to include *sins against the spirit.* These include the invisible sins of fear (anxiety and worry), accusation (judgment, envy, comparison), lack of joy in the Father, bitterness and unforgiveness, and many others that I have not discussed, such as guilt, self-hatred and self-rejection, self-pity, idolatry (including intellectual idolatry), and many more. You will see in the next few chapters how these sins against the spirit can directly affect our health.

Chapter 3

Puzzle Piece #2 of 3: The Body's Design

Many of God's commands are designed to protect us from disease. For example, sexual fidelity prevents the spread of sexually transmitted diseases. Through the careful handling and removal of corpses, quarantine of those infected with disease, and separation and sanitation in childbirth, we are also protected from disease. An excellent book titled *None of These Diseases,* coauthored by Dr. S.I. McMillen, M.D., and his grandson, Dr. David E. Stern, M.D., describes the health benefits of many of God's commands. For example, God commanded the Israelites to locate their latrine outside of the camp and cover up their "business" with a shovel (Deut 23:12-13). This prevented the spread of disease. The book explains how the cholera epidemic in England in the mid-1800's was fueled by open sewage in the streets. It killed over 150,000 people and later gave cause to build what has evolved into today's modern waste treatment systems. If they had done it God's way, then that epidemic would not have occurred.

These are examples of the completeness of God's commands. He does not give us a reason for why He does what he does. Sometimes we understand it at a later time, and sometimes we never understand it. I think it's healthy to recognize that when He gives a command, it is not necessarily for our spiritual well-being only. Often there are physical benefits as well.

> *When God gives a command, it is not necessarily for our spiritual well-being only. Often there are physical benefits as well.*

In this chapter, I want to look at some basic biology of the human body. I am not a medical professional, and, as noted earlier, I am not giving you any medical advice. My purpose is to give those in the body of Christ a fresh and biblical perspective on disease. As far as the treatment of a given disease is concerned, I have previously advised you to look to the Lord and seek His wisdom first and above all else. The Lord wants to bless you with wisdom, and He wants to fellowship with you. "In all your ways acknowledge Him, and he will make your path straight" (Prov 3:6). All medical decisions are fully your responsibility.

Now let's look at some basic human anatomy and physiology. The human body has two primary controlling systems. The first is the central nervous system (CNS). Basically, the CNS governs how the five senses—touch, taste, hearing, sight, and smell—receive stimuli, process it, and then respond. The second controlling system is the internal chemistry of the body, called the endocrine system. The CNS operates with rapid electrochemical impulses. The endocrine system, by contrast, responds with slower chemical or hormonal changes in the body. The two systems overlap and are intimately integrated.

The body's chemical composition is action-packed and in a constant state of change. The normal state of chemical balance for the body is known as *homeostasis*. During times of stress, even anticipated stress, the body's chemistry changes but still operates within expected and measurable parameters for that particular activity—for example, sports activities or childbirth—and that condition is called *allostasis*. This chemical balance is established by the nine endocrine glands: the pituitary, thyroid, parathyroid, adrenal, pineal, thymus, pancreas, and gonad glands (ovaries and testes). The ninth gland is the hypothalamus, which is unique because of its neural integration. This is known as a *neuroendocrine* gland.

The Endocrine System

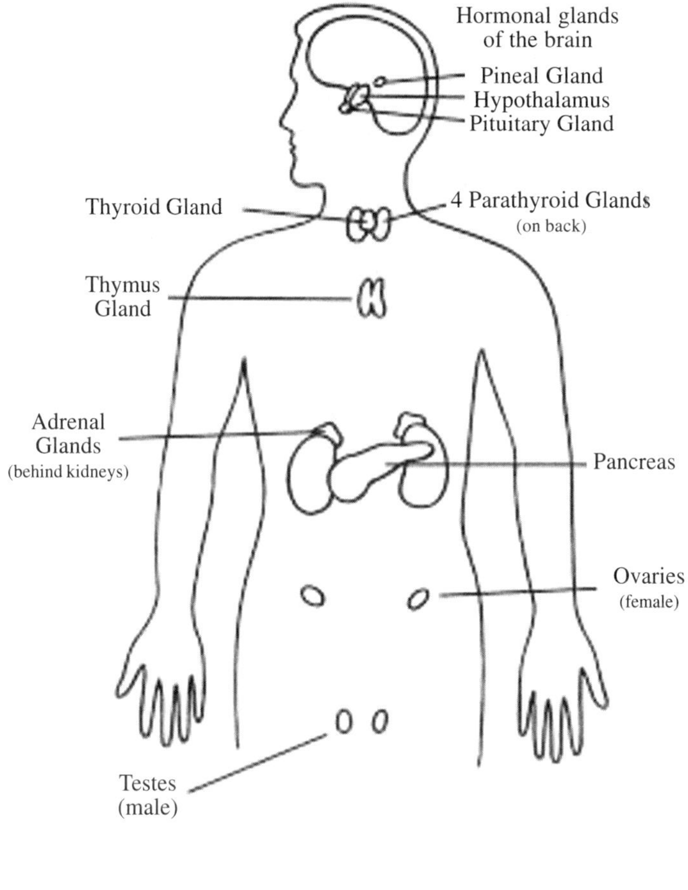

The endocrine system and its chemical functions affect virtually every system of the body. The skeletal, muscular, nervous, cardiovascular, lymphatic, respiratory, digestive, urinary, reproductive, and integumentary (skin and hair) systems are all integrated at one level or another with hormonal activity.

There are too many hormones and combinations of hormones to list here. What is important to note is that, when the body is out of balance for extended periods due to over-secretion or under-secretion of hormones, there is a higher likelihood of disease.

The Endocrine System

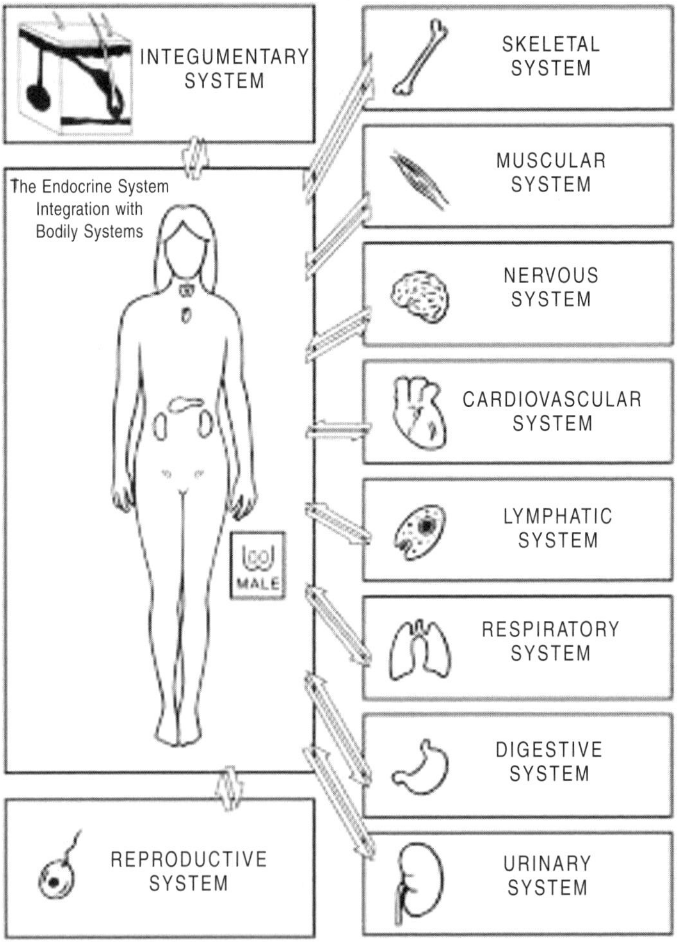

The hormones of the endocrine system are regulated through two different stimuli. One is glandular and relatively automatic. For example, blood chemistry is continuously monitored by the body and adjusted without conscious thought. The second method is through conscious and unconscious CNS stimulation. For example, the outside temperature may rise and generate the hormonal response for hot weather, and within a few minutes you're sweating. Or there may be conscious stimulation, such as a wife telling her husband, "Honey, we're going to be late to the game, and you're going to miss the first quarter." The husband's adrenal glands awaken, and he has the energy to speed up. These chemical changes are infinitely complex. But what's important to understand is that our bodies are not strictly mechanical. We can change our own body chemistry with thoughts, whether we recognize it or not.

We can change our body chemistry with thought.

Medical researchers Andrew Schally of Poland and Roger Guillemin of France worked independently on identical projects that won them each a Nobel Prize in medicine in 1977. Their work showed that the hormonal secretions of the hypothalamus gland and its direct connection to the pituitary gland are vital to the operation of the entire endocrine system. Thus, the hypothalamus gland is considered the master gland of the endocrine system, or the computer control center of the body's hormonal chemistry. The hypothalamus is located in the middle of the brain. This design is vital from a spiritual point of view. Satan and his army are very experienced and fully aware of the design of the human body. They know how to strategically attack it, instigating a disease in us when we are unaware. Let me explain further.

Medical researcher Hans Selye is generally recognized as the founder of endocrinology. He was born in Vienna, Austria, in 1907 and died in Montreal, Canada, in 1982. He was a physician, author, and professor, but he is most famous for his work on what is called the

General Adaptation Syndrome (GAS), which many believe should have won him a Nobel Prize in medicine.

The GAS details the hormonal changes that the human body goes through as a result of stress, both good and bad kinds. These are detailed in Selye's book, *The Stress of Life*. To summarize, his model includes three stages. The first stage is the *alarm reaction*, a fight-or-flight response to circumstances. Second is the *stage of resistance*, in which long-term metabolic adjustments occur in the body. Third is the *stage of exhaustion*, which is characterized by the collapse of vital bodily systems.

STAGES OF THE GENERAL ADAPTATION SYNDROME

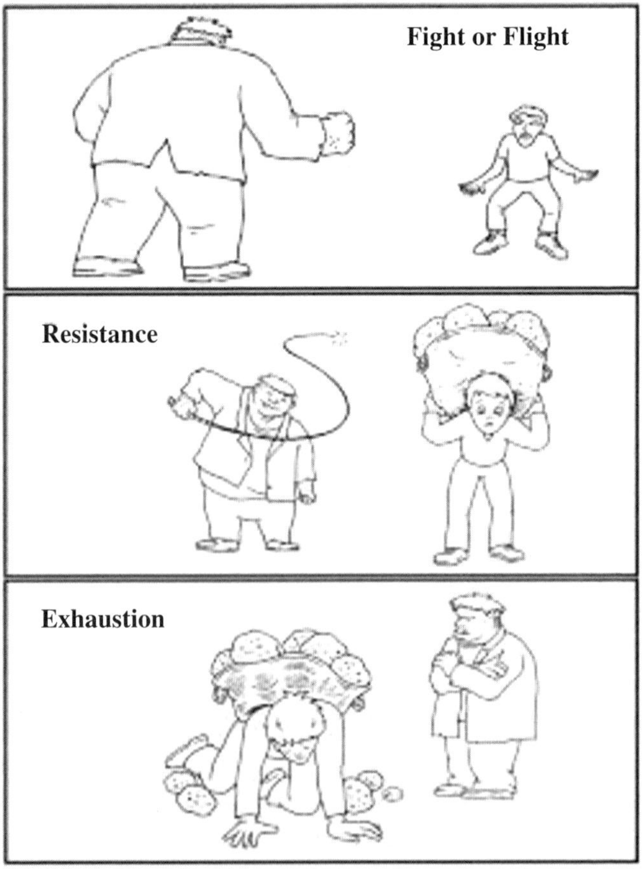

The alarm phase can occur in a number of different ways on a practical level. A person might be scared of having a car wreck because surrounding drivers are driving at seventy-five miles per hour on the freeway, or a woman might be afraid of making her husband unhappy because he yells at her every day, and sometimes she worries that he might hit her. Or perhaps an employee can't stand his tyrant boss, whose primary management technique is intimidation and confrontation; every day the employee is afraid of losing his job. In the alarm phase, the body produces high amounts of adrenaline (or *epinephrine*, to use the American term). This in turn starts a complex series of events that I can only summarize. While in the alarm phase, and while in fear, your digestion and immune systems become inhibited (specifically, your white blood cell production dramatically decreases). The blood's clotting ability increases, along with memory and pain threshold. Also, an individual will not have any sexual interest during this phase.

While in fear your digestion and immune systems become inhibited. Your body's blood clotting abilities increase along with your memory and pain threshold.

The second stage, the resistance phase, is equally complex. The body attempts to reestablish homeostasis in the body with the resources it has, until those resources become exhausted. This phase can last months or years. There may be permanent alterations in the body chemistry in this stage.

In the final stage, the exhaustion phase, we see a disease develop with the breakdown of the bodily system.

Hopefully, you can see from the GAS that the emotion of fear, and more generally stress, when it has a long-term presence in your life, can be detrimental to your health.

In response to stress, the body secretes cortisol, a *glucocorticoid* hormone that is often referred to as the *stress hormone*. Cortisol is activated by the endocrine system's adrenal glands. Its mere presence is not detrimental to the body; in fact, the adrenaline/cortisol balance is important in the regulation of the entire body. However, cortisol becomes detrimental when the level of the hormone is raised and remains at chronically high levels. At that point, it can affect virtually every system in the body and can lead to a gradual deterioration of health.

The book *The Cortisol Connection* by Shawn Talbott, Ph.D., contains an excellent and easy-to-read description of cortisol-induced health conditions, such as obesity, heart disease, depression, diabetes, osteoporosis, suppressed libido, immune system suppression, and more. Talbott writes from a nutritional perspective and gives fundamentally sound advice. However, his is a secular book that does not discuss the spiritual dimension of our lives. I mention it because of its biological information. The author makes an interesting comment: "Because the brain is so well developed, it can also respond to imagined stress with the very same stress response that is supposed to be reserved for life-or-death (fight-or-flight) situations" (p. 32). Basically, the body cannot distinguish between what is real and what is imagined. This can be seen in the fact that the body has the same physiological response to sexual fantasy as it does to reality. We also have the capacity to cultivate fear and bitterness from imagined scenarios and beliefs that are not real or accurate. In the next chapter, I will discuss our spiritual battle, and you will see how Satan is the father of lies and how he can introduce these thoughts into our minds.[2]

The brain cannot distinguish between reality and fantasy. Therefore the body responds the same to imagined stress as it does to genuine life-or-death situations.

[2] Another excellent book that gives a detailed description of the body's endocrine response from a biological perspective is *Why Zebras Don't Get Ulcers* by Robert M. Sapolsky. However, this is secular biology and does not discuss matters from a biblically holistic perspective.

Think for a moment about the consequences of fear and anxiety. What will your health be like in five years if you have inhibited digestion? Will you have a colon disease? What will be the condition of your health as a result of heightened clotting or thickened blood? Will you have circulatory problems? What might happen if you suffer from an inhibited immune system, after you have lived under the stress of fear for an extended period of time?

Your cells undergo millions of divisions each day. When cells do not divide correctly, they are programmed to self-destruct. This is called *apoptosis.* Some cells do not self-destruct and yet do not pose any threat to the body. However, carcinogens and other unknown influences can cause cells to mutate into a variety of types of harmful cancer cells. Our wonderful neuro-oncologist, Dr. Virginia Stark-Vance, told us that the National Cancer Institute has determined that the average American is faced with harmful cancer cells an average of two hundred times in their lifetime. Did you know that you've had cancer cells in your body on numerous occasions? What happens to these cells? Well, if you're healthy, your immune system has done what God has designed it to do and has attacked the cells and removed them before they manifested themselves. But what if your immune system is compromised by fear and anxiety? God has already instructed us what we should do with that fear and anxiety (see 1 Peter 5:7).

I can provide multiple examples of people who should be healthy but are battling cancer. Certainly my hypothesis does not explain every situation, but I wonder how many have a compromised immune system. When I had this discussion with one dear friend, the Lord opened his eyes, and he began to see a host of issues that had created long-term anxiety in his life to the point that he could not sleep and had to go to the doctor for medication. He began to see how his body's own immune system had become compromised due to anxiety. Praise God and the work of the Holy Spirit for opening his spiritual eyes. As of this writing, he is healthy and cancer-free. His faith has grown, and he has taken to heart a key biblical principal: "Do not be anxious about anything, but in everything, by prayer and petition, with thanksgiving present your requests to God" (Phil 4:6, NASB).

Now let's take this discussion to another level. It has been proven that through the General Adaptation Syndrome, fear alters body chemistry and is most detrimental to one's health over an extended period of time. What about other sins of the spirit, such as guilt? Can it, too, change one's body chemistry? What about bitterness and unforgiveness, or the host of other negative emotions? If so, can it be said that guilt *always* leads to a specific disease? Is this study that specific? And what about positive emotions? Do they benefit health?

I'm not aware of any medical study that tracks disease based on emotions. If researchers could scientifically track a specific emotion to a specific disease, then that emotion could be identified as a *signature stressor*. I have not found anyone who has made this link in every situation; the body is too complex. However, Christian author Don Colbert, M.D., has written an excellent book, *Deadly Emotions*, that discusses the fundamentals of this specific subject and makes some excellent recommendations. I believe that all the negative emotions generate changes in our body chemistry on one level or another. Some people have bodies that are more sensitive to these changes than others. However, since the human body is incredibly complex and the number of variables so large, it's virtually impossible to track specific emotions to specific diseases. The possible outcomes are so great that they are indeterminable.

What about the reverse situation? Do positive emotions help our health? In the book *Why Men Don't Listen and Women Can't Read Maps*, authors Barbara and Allan Pease note that an amorous interlude for a man increases testosterone levels, which in turn fortifies bones and muscles. The hormone DHEA (dehydroepiandrosterone) is released, which improves cognition and builds the immune system.

In addition, endorphins are released in the brain. For women, the estrogen release increases bone mass and improves the cardiovascular system. So yes, it's true, more loving sex as God has designed it (i.e., with positive emotion) results in better health and longer life.

Another book you should consider reading, and one which I can give my highest recommendation, is Pastor Henry Wright's book, *A More Excellent Way*. Pastor Wright and his staff at Pleasant Valley Church in Thomaston, Georgia, have perhaps the most successful healing ministry in the world. In addition to the book, they offer phone counseling and monthly conferences. In over twenty years of ministry, Pastor Wright has kept records of the people he has ministered to and their diseases and what he has determined to be the spiritual root causes. His work would not fulfill the research standards required by the academic or medical communities, but on a practical level where "the proof is in the pudding," Pastor Wright is correct an extremely high percentage of the time. In his book, he lists over sixty diseases and describes what he considers the spiritual root causes. These are the trends or tendencies that he has recognized. I prefer to think of the book as his pastoral recommendation to me as a layperson in the church. I do not agree with all that Pastor Wright teaches, and it's not realistic to expect everyone in the body of Christ to agree perfectly. But I do have the highest level of respect and love for him and his ministry and the staff at Pleasant Valley Church. He is passionate in his love for the Lord!

In summary, our body chemistry is the second of three complex concepts that combine to cause disease in the life of a saint. The first puzzle piece broadens the definition of sin to include the forgotten invisible sins against the spirit. The second piece shows that our body chemistry is altered by thought through the endocrine system, and that altered chemistry, or chemical imbalance, can result in disease. In the next chapter, I will turn to the subject of our spiritual battle. This final piece of the puzzle will allow us to see the whole picture.

Chapter 4

Puzzle Piece #3 of 3: Our Spiritual Battle

Most Christians in America seem to believe that we live in spiritually neutral territory. After all, my life is very comfortable; I live just two miles from a Wal-Mart Supercenter, Sam's Wholesale Club, a Super Target, and a Chick-Fil-A. Life just doesn't get any better than that, right? If my physical life is so filled with material comforts, why should my spiritual life be any different? Well, unfortunately, that is not biblically-based thinking. In this chapter, I'd like to take a closer look at our spiritual battle.

Scriptures tell us that this world offers temptation in the form of lust of the eyes, lust of the flesh and the boastful pride of life (1 John 2:16). Given the opportunity, sin grows from that point to have a greater and greater place in our life. In the context of disease I am not referring to a spiritual battle in its initial stages. I am referring to a sin issue and spiritual battle that has been on going for many years and has time to manifest physically. It is from that perspective that I write this chapter.

Have you ever thought about what you would see if you could see right now with spiritual eyes? What activity would you see going on around you? Would you see guardian angels, or your loved ones who have preceded you in death? Would you see anyone in that great cloud of witnesses mentioned in Hebrews 12:1? Perhaps you would see fallen angels. What are all those fallen angels doing right now, anyway? Are they in a celestial paradise somewhere having a beach party? Are there any in your city or neighborhood, perhaps even in your home? How many fallen angels are there? A hundred? A thousand? A million? Well, let's take a closer look at Scripture so that we can answer these questions and gain a biblical perspective.

First, let's review a series of scriptures that may seem unrelated. I provide them for some basic information about who is who and who is where in this world and in heaven. Currently, our Father is in heaven sitting on the throne. The Scriptures tell us that Jesus is at the right hand of

God the Father, both sitting (Col 3:1) and standing (Acts 7:55). The Holy Spirit was sent to us (John 14:16-17) and resides in this world with us as our helper and comforter. As a whole, mankind has dominion over this world (Gen 1:26). However, the saints in the church are actually living in conflict with this world (John 15:18-19) and are not made for this world, for it is ultimately not our home (Heb 13:14). Of course, we are made to worship God and fellowship with Him in our eternal home.

There was a time when Satan had authority in heaven, but he was removed from his position (Isa 14:12). He is now considered to be god of this world (2 Cor 4:4). So it is most likely that all the members of his kingdom are focused on his work here on this planet, with the exception of those who have been bound for now and will be released in the end times (Rev 9:15). Satan continues to have access to the throne of our heavenly Father (Job 1) and is continuously accusing the saints (Rev 12:10). He has also been given the title of "Prince of the power of the air" (Eph 2:2). This is harmonious with Luke 11:24, which tells of evil spirits being cast into the "dry place." I do not think this refers to the actual air we breathe, but to the invisible spirit world that is around us here on this planet. It may seem as if Satan's kingdom is in the air because his kingdom is made up of spirits that are not bound by the law of gravity or other laws of nature. Satan also has the power of death (Heb 2:14), but he must get permission before he may use it (Rev 1:18 and Job 2:6).

Satan has a plan of his own for this world, which is in opposition to the gospel. He desires to "steal, kill, and destroy" (John 10:10). He is the "father of lies" (John 8:44), and he even masquerades as an "angel of light" (2 Cor 11:14). One way that he occupies himself is by roaming around the earth looking for someone to devour (1 Pet 5:8), and that is exactly what he was doing in Job 1:7 when he began his dialogue with God regarding Job.

In Luke 22:31, Satan demanded permission to "sift" the apostle Peter "like wheat." He is not omniscient, omnipresent, or omnipotent—only God is that—but he is the commander of an innumerably large company of fallen angels that make it seem as though he is everywhere at once. He does not know exactly what we are thinking, but he and his workers have had thousands of years of experience understanding human behavior.

The Scriptures refer to the *kingdom* of darkness. So what is a kingdom? Have you ever visited Manhattan in New York City? While in the plane and on your approach into the airport, you can look down and see that jungle of skyscrapers. The population of Manhattan at night is around seven million, and during a business day, it's over twelve million. That's a lot of people! They each have their own careers, relationships, and families. They are of different nationalities and work in every industry you can imagine. Some are tall, some are short, some are men, and some are women. There are senior citizens and members of every age group, all the way down to newborn infants. And all that activity is going on just in Manhattan, one of five boroughs in New York City.

The kingdom of darkness is a similarly busy place. There is much planning and coordination of efforts. Directives are issued all the way down the administrative chain. Currently the population of the earth is more than six billion. It's reasonable to guess that there are billions and billions of fallen angels under the directive of Satan and his organization. At least, it's accurate to say that there are plenty of fallen angels to go around. (I use the term *fallen angel* to refer loosely to any member of the kingdom of darkness. For my purposes, that term is synonymous with demons, evil spirits, unclean spirits, unholy angels, and devils. They are all agents for Satan and his kingdom.)

The message of Ephesians 6:10-12 is most commonly read from a kingdom perspective:

> *Finally, be strong in the Lord and in the strength of His might. Put on the full armor of God, so that you will be able to stand firm against the schemes of the devil. For our struggle is not against flesh and blood, but against the rulers, against the powers, against the world forces of this darkness, against the spiritual forces of wickedness in the heavenly places.* (NASB)

When I read that passage, it tells me that yes, there are Satanic schemes and many participants in his organization, ranging all the way from his command central—which is probably orchestrating world governments and the activities of the false religions of the world—down to the persecution of individual saints in the church.

Hopefully by now I have convinced you that we as saints live in enemy territory, despite the material comforts that we enjoy. I began this book by explaining how I discovered a lack of teaching in this area. I have read Ephesians 6 countless times, but it never became meaningful to me until I thought of it in the context of disease. Formerly, if you had asked me to discuss the work of Satan, I would have told you that there were many evil spirits in third-world countries, such as Haiti or Ethiopia. I could have told you of extreme situations in this country, but I could not have given you an everyday example of Ephesians 6 in my life or my family's. I couldn't have guessed how Satan might execute his plan to steal someone's health. I will elaborate on that plan in this chapter and build on it in the next.

> *The primary focal point of Satan's scheming attack is on the minds of the saints.*

The primary focal point of Satan's scheming attack is on the minds of the saints. Let me show you three convincing verses. First is Genesis 3:8-11:

> *Then the man and his wife heard the sound of the LORD God as he was walking in the garden in the cool of the day, and they hid from the LORD God among the trees of the garden. But the LORD God called to the man, "Where are you?"*
>
> *He answered, "I heard you in the garden, and I was afraid because I was naked; so I hid."*
>
> *And he said, "Who told you that you were naked? Have you eaten from the tree that I commanded you not to eat from?"* (NASB)

The most fascinating verse in this passage is verse 11: "*Who* told you . . . ?" God is asking Adam "Who," not "How" or "What." There were only two people created at that moment, Adam and Eve, and they were being asked the question. Who else could it be? Could it be the snake? I'm willing to bet that the snake was no longer in the area, so allow me to speculate for a moment.

Prior to the fall of man, Adam and Eve enjoyed unbroken fellowship with the Father. They had no sin, and there was no separation; they could have lived eternally! But with that sin, man's spirit became separated from the Father. Prior to the fall, I don't think that the members of Satan's kingdom could approach Adam or Eve on a spiritual level. They were off-limits in the Garden. Again, I am speculating, yet I believe they had to be approached on a physical level, which is why Satan chose to channel his voice through the serpent. He was not permitted to enter the minds of Adam and Eve. After the fall, however, for the first time Adam and Eve began to *hear the thoughts* of Satan's kingdom. It was an attack on their minds. Thus, God the Father said, "*Who* told you . . ." *Who in Satan's kingdom told you this?*

Let me show this to you again, this time in the New Testament in Matthew 16:13-23:

> *Now when Jesus came into the district of Caesarea Philippi, He was asking His disciples, "Who do people say that the Son of Man is?"*
>
> *And they said, "Some say John the Baptist; and others, Elijah; but still others, Jeremiah, or one of the prophets."*
>
> *He said to them, "But who do you say that I am?"*
>
> *Simon Peter answered, "You are the Christ, the Son of the living God."*
>
> *And Jesus said to him, "Blessed are you, Simon Barjona, because flesh and blood did not reveal this to you, but My Father who is in heaven. I also say to you that you are Peter, and upon this rock I will build My church; and the gates of Hades will not overpower it. I will give you the keys of the kingdom of heaven; and whatever you bind on earth shall have been bound in heaven, and whatever you loose on earth shall have been loosed in heaven." Then He warned the disciples that they should tell no one that He was the Christ.*
>
> *From that time Jesus began to show His disciples that He must go to Jerusalem, and suffer many things from the elders and chief priests and scribes, and be killed, and be raised up on the third day. Peter took Him aside and began to rebuke Him,*

> *saying, "God forbid it, Lord! This shall never happen to You."*
>
> *But He turned and said to Peter, "Get behind Me, Satan! You are a stumbling block to Me; for you are not setting your mind on God's interests, but man's."* (NASB)

Here, everything occurs in one chapter. First, in verses 13 and 14, Jesus asks the disciples, Peter included, "Who do the people think I am?" The people use their own power of reasoning to conclude that He is a prophet, such as Jeremiah, Elijah, or John the Baptist. This is the first source of thoughts that man has: his own reasoning. Then, in verse 15, Jesus asks Peter directly, "Who do you say I am?" and Peter responds with tremendous words of faith: "You are the Christ, the Son of the Living God." Wow! A fellow could only make a statement like that through the enlightenment of the Father. Peter was speaking thoughts revealed by God the Father. The Holy Spirit, who lives in every believer, is the second source of thoughts that man can hear. Sometimes these thoughts come more in the form of promptings.

Now let's jump down to verse 23. Jesus has just given Peter one of the most wonderful compliments anyone could ever hope to receive in verse 18. But in verses 21 and 22, Peter tries to stop Jesus from teaching about his upcoming suffering. Jesus turns to him not five verses after complimenting him and says, right to Peter's face, "Get behind me, Satan!" Wow again! It looks like Peter may not be so special after all. Here we see the third source of thoughts. These are thoughts from the kingdom of darkness flowing through Peter. All three categories are revealed in eleven verses: the thoughts of man, the thoughts of God, and the thoughts of Satan.

> *All believers can hear thoughts from three sources:*
> 1) *Our own minds,*
> 2) *Our Father in heaven, and*
> 3) *Satan's Kingdom.*

One thing that made Peter special was that he was so typically human. He was passionate and stubborn. He was wrong on many occasions; he even argued with Paul in Acts. And he had the education of a sailor. Sounds like he belongs in my family! Some interpret the statement in verse 18, "Upon this rock I will build my church," as referring not to Peter individually, but to Peter as the representative of ordinary men. I don't disagree with that interpretation. From the time of Christ, God no longer used the priests as his representatives, but rather established a personal relationship with men so they could be His vessels in this world and form His Church.

Let me give you one final verse addressing the world of thought (2 Cor 10:3-6):

> *For though we walk in the flesh, we do not war after the flesh: (For the weapons of our warfare are not carnal, but mighty through God to the pulling down of strongholds;) Casting down imaginations, and every high thing that exalts itself against the knowledge of God, and bringing into captivity every thought to the obedience of Christ; And having in a readiness to revenge all disobedience, when your obedience is fulfilled.* (KJV)

Paul tells us in verse 3 that we are fighting a spiritual battle. What is a "high thing" in verse 5 that can exalt itself against the knowledge of God? There are many opinions about what this means, because it is a seldom-used word. I've concluded that the language refers to a person, because only a person can think and actually make the decision to exalt himself against the knowledge of God. If it were in fact a person, then it would either be a human, a righteous angel (and a righteous angel would not be opposing the knowledge of God), or a fallen angel. Even if the verse does not refer to an evil spirit directly, it does so indirectly, since all that opposes the knowledge of God originates from Satan on one level or another.

Paul is fully aware that we can receive thoughts from Satan's kingdom. The context of this verse is spiritual warfare (v. 3), which is why he tells us to bring all our thoughts into obedience. He knows what we are up against.

What is a "stronghold" in the spiritual context of this verse? This word can probably mean several things. Again, since the context is spiritual warfare, the definition can include the coordinated effort of two or more evil spirits that are harassing a saint. This is an area of our lives in which Satan's agents have set up an area of control, perhaps in the form of thought patterns or habits that are unbiblical. The verse also states that these strongholds can be torn down using our spiritual weapons.

I am not saying that Satan and his fallen angels do our thinking. Certainly not! We are free moral agents, and we can choose to think what we want; this is the essence of free will. But Satan's army has the ability to give us thoughts. Even Jesus faced temptation and turned Satan away in favor of God's truth. With every temptation, Jesus responded with a verse from the Word of God. We have the same choice: to receive, believe, and establish Satan's lies in our lives, or to receive, believe, and establish the truth of God. To draw a high-tech analogy, each of us is like a computer with a constant connection to the Internet, being probed regularly by hackers looking to do damage to our computer. Once Satan finds an opening, he can plant a seed and open a channel that will lead to the eventual downfall of our biological hard drive, much like a hacker can plant a computer virus. As I stated when I began this chapter, most Christians in America seem to believe we live in spiritually neutral territory, so they never give this much thought.

Now let's dig deeper. We know that Satan's army can give us thoughts. We know that if we don't turn them away and if we believe the lies of Satan, then we are establishing Satan's kingdom in that area of our life. So what else do we need to know about the work of evil spirits? First, I would point out that Jesus believed in evil spirits. My personal study revealed that in nearly one-third of the instances in which Jesus healed someone, he also cast out an evil spirit. In Luke 9:1-2, he sent out the twelve disciples and gave them authority over all the demons and to heal diseases. Then he sent them to proclaim the Kingdom of God. Then again in Luke 10, he sent out the seventy in pairs to heal the sick and proclaim the Kingdom of God. When they came back, they were "full of joy and saying even the demons were subject to us in your name" (v. 17).

A critical distinction needs to be made in the church today. There is a difference between spiritual *possession* (the Greek term is *daimonizomai, Strong's* #1139) that automatically jumps into everyone's mind, and spiritual *oppression.* The biggest distinction here is that a Christian cannot be possessed. I repeat, Christians *cannot be possessed!* However, they can certainly be *oppressed.* Evil spirit activity does not resemble the portrayals of Hollywood. The first thing that comes to mind is the film *The Exorcist.* The second is the cartoons we've all seen over the years, such as *Casper* or *Scooby Doo.* I disagree with the way spirits are portrayed in both. I do not believe that there is an evil spirit in every closet, waiting to growl at me like a dog or make my head spin around.

I also disagree with the churches that choose to avoid the topic altogether and never equip their flock to recognize spiritual oppression. It is unfortunate, yet I believe that Satan's army can come and go freely in some churches today, completely unnoticed and unopposed. I have met those in church leadership who could not recognize spiritual oppression or even the most obvious presence of an evil spirit or his work. They are even less equipped to respond to the situation in a biblical manner. This type of leadership offers little training in this subject area. If you want to stir up a hornet's nest, go to a church that avoids teaching on evil spirits and avoids the passages concerning spiritual warfare; these churches are numerous and common. Tell them that evil spirits are active and present in their lives and in their homes, bringing hardship upon them. Show me those in that church with diseases, and I will find a large percentage that are living with spiritual oppression and in partnership with Satan's army in some area of their lives.

The apostle Paul believed in evil spirit oppression. We don't have the full details regarding his "thorn in the flesh," which he refers to in 2 Corinthian 12, but he does call it a "messenger from Satan." The word *messenger* is a noun meaning "a person bringing a message." Angels commonly serve as messengers. In the case of Paul, there is much debate, but it is reasonable to conclude that the messenger was a fallen angel from Satan who laid claim to Paul, or a physical affliction wrought by the hand of Satan, as in the case of Job. Paul lived with spiritual and/or physical oppression in an area of his life, and since he said the reason was to "keep him from exalting himself," it is reasonable to conclude that his personal sin had to do with pride.

The body of Christ is empowered to respond to this activity of Satan. In 1 Corinthians 12:10, one of the gifts of the Spirit is "distinguishing of spirits" (NASB). This is not something that everyone is able to do. The Holy Spirit orchestrates the activities of those in the body of Christ, and each disciple has a purpose and role, whether as a teacher, administrator, minister, or prayer warrior.

I can't tell you how impressed I was when I read about one large congregation that fasted every Monday, with voluntary participation in a solid food fast, for those who had asked for prayer or healing. I have grown to view fasting as highly regarded in the Kingdom of God and as particularly relevant to spiritual warfare.

Many called and supported us during Teresa's illness, asking, "What can I do?" Well, there wasn't much to do in the actual care of Teresa.

Instead, I would ask them to fast for her. It was a sacrificial act rooted in love. Of all those who asked, those people in the body of Christ who fasted and prayed for Teresa were a tremendous blessing to us, especially toward the end of her life.

I want to give you examples of evil spirit activity in today's world, but I must also tell you in advance that my examples will be relatively boring by design. I am writing to the ordinary believer. Yes, I can tell you extreme stories, like that of a fellow widower with whom I have become friends, whose wife was diagnosed with sixty-two personalities and eventually took her own life. Yes, I believe that she was greatly oppressed with evil spirits. But theirs was an extreme case. What about Joe Average Christian? Let me give you testimony from my own life.

I have already told you of my battle with bitterness in my discussion of sin. There was a day when I was driving to pick up some supplies for my business. It was a troublesome task to find the supplies, and I became frustrated after spending nearly two hours on the phone. Now I was driving for over two hours to pick them up. All this time, we were turning away business because the machine that needed the supplies was not operational without the product. Well, I was tense and began to get angry. Then it escalated, and my anger and bitterness began to boil. I was under spiritual attack. Satan's guys were feeding me ideas, and I wasn't taking any of them captive. I don't know what was going on in my body chemistry, but I'm sure it wasn't good for my health.

Then, driving past a shopping center, I observed an older couple leisurely walking together into a grocery store. I noticed the tree branches blowing peacefully in the light breeze. I love trees. I can name all the trees native to my area, and my favorite vacation was to Yosemite National Park to see the giant Sequoias. Talk about the glory of God—you need to see those trees! Then I noticed the cheerful birds whistling, just like in a Disney film. Finally, it hit me: *Klay, the anger and bitterness are your problem.* Everyone else—the older couple, the trees, the birds—all seemed to be fine. If you could have seen my brain on the inside, I'm sure it would have looked like a piece of steel wool all knotted up.

I knew something was up but didn't know what it was; this occurred before my wife's illness and before we had received any teaching on the subject. So I prayed out loud in desperation: "Father, make it go away!" I knew that if I resisted Satan, he would flee from me (James 4:7). My prayer might not have been technically correct, but the Spirit interceded for me (Rom 8:26). Shortly after I prayed, I reached my destination, bought my supplies, and got in my truck for the return trip. I had the most peaceful drive home. My machine at the store was still not operating, and I was still losing money. Nevertheless, the drive was very pleasant. The bitterness had gone from me, and I was relaxed, singing a song. That is the Kingdom of God—"Righteousness, joy, and peace in the Holy Spirit" (Rom 14:17)—and I was enjoying His peace. Satan's attack had been thwarted with a promise from the Word of God.

Has this happened to you? The scenario is not dramatic. I know some churches will never teach on this subject for fear of being labeled as extremist or fanatical. No one will ever make a movie about my story. But it serves as an example of a normal day-to-day battle of the spirit. This battle could have escalated if I had failed to recognize it and allowed it to manifest. There are many examples in the Scriptures of how small battles turned into major strongholds in people's lives. For example, the man in the tombs that had many evil spirits (Mark 5) most likely did not start out with all his issues. They probably built up one by one until Satan's forces had him cornered. It was probably the same with Mary Magdalene, who had seven evil spirits (Luke 8). Evil spirits are just as active today as they were in Jesus' day. The only difference is that we don't want to recognize them or have grown too smart for our own good, explaining them away with medical diagnoses or other logical rationalizations. But Scripture reveals that Satan's armies of fallen angels are around us and are proactive in doing Satan's work, even in our own homes. There are plenty of them to go around. I pray that you will not get caught unaware.

This concludes the third of three complex factors that combine to cause disease in the life of a saint. In the first part, we broadened the definition of sin to include the sins against the spirit. In the next chapter, we examined our bodies' physiological response to fear and other emotions. In this chapter, we have looked at how Satan and his army of evil spirits can attack a saint and bring about spiritual oppression. In the next chapter, I will combine all three concepts to show you the whole picture.

CHAPTER 5

THE PUZZLE COMPLETED: EXPOSING SATAN'S STRATEGY

I'd like to review for a moment before I pull all the pieces together. I believe that God still heals people. However, healing is not the focus of this book. My primary goals are to prevent disease before it occurs and to give a solid biblical response to disease when it does occur.

In Chapter 1, I listed the seven reasons for disease that I found in my study of Scripture. Of those seven, there are three to which we can respond: disease caused by our own sin, disease caused by the sin of our ancestral fathers, and disease caused by the sin of others. In chapters 2, 3, and 4, I discussed three seemingly unrelated topics: the sins of the spirit, the body's response to stress, and our spiritual battle. These three chapters, when understood as a whole, explain how our own sin could cause a disease.

First I clarified that sin includes the invisible sins against the spirit, such as fear, unforgiveness, and bitterness, to name a few. Next, I discussed the basics of human physiology and described the endocrine system. I explained how the body responds during times of stress, both real and imagined, as detailed in the General Adaptation Syndrome. This is scientific proof that our bodies experience a physiological response to emotion. Many of those emotions arise because of sins against the spirit. In the fourth chapter, I talked about our spiritual battle and how Satan strategically attacks our minds. In essence, what I have done is uncover the link from the spirit to the mind, and then to the body. This is commonly referred to as the spirit-mind-body connection.

These explanations will not cover all diseases. However, in my opinion they do explain a majority of the diseases touching the lives of believers in the church today. Almost everyone with a disease can determine its cause by asking the Lord to reveal it to them, and by seeking wise counsel from their church leaders. In addition, I believe that when the sin issue is removed, there is a possibility of healing, because God has designed our bodies to heal themselves.

Now let me pull together the puzzle pieces of chapters 2, 3, and 4. First, realize that Satan's plan, like that of the hacker within your computer, is invisible. Satan works at the spiritual level. We know from Scripture that Satan is roaming around like a roaring lion looking for someone to devour (1 Peter 5:8). Although Scripture states that *Satan* is roaming around, it's also fair to conclude that we face persecution from his followers as well, the fallen angels. We have also seen how Satan has the ability to give us thoughts. We are tempted in our thoughts first, but just because we have a thought it does not mean that we are in sin. A single thought is not sin. We know that even Jesus was tempted. But we are commanded to take every thought captive, to meditate on God's Word and to resist Satan. We can follow Jesus' example and recite Scripture when we are tempted. However, we don't always remember to do this—or worse, we choose not to.

One thought turns into another thought. Pretty soon, these thoughts become a mentality, or a whole thought process. Then we truly believe what we are thinking, and we start speaking it! Some scholars believe that this is what the Bible calls a "stronghold." At that point, we have bought into a lie from Satan's kingdom and accepted it as truth. As we verbalize and act on this lie, the thoughts begin to manifest and become evident in our lives in a manner that is not biblically based. Additional examples of these thoughts that can affect our health include guilt, self-hatred, jealousy, comparison, and lack of joy in our Father, just to name a few. Our heavenly Father has a hedge of protection around us, but as we verbalize and establish Satan's kingdom in our lives, we remove ourselves from the protection of our heavenly Father. Satan accuses us before the throne. Our heavenly Father is patient and longsuffering. However, there comes a time, as determined by Him, that we must face the consequence of our actions. Many times that consequence is a disease.

> *It is Satan's plan to attack our minds so that we think ourselves (and often times eat ourselves) into a disease.*

Now the spirit-mind-body connection is clear to see. After the spiritual attack on our thoughts, our thoughts can, through our endocrine system, actually alter our body chemistry. This can occur subtly or dramatically. It begins with the hypothalamus gland, the neuroendocrine gland of the endocrine system that is located in the center of the brain. From there, the message has the potential to spread to every major system of the body. Referring back to the General Adaptation Syndrome discussed by Dr. Hans Selye in *The Stress of Life,* this has been proven medically. The body undergoes three phases of response, and after a sustained period, which is different for everyone, the body breaks down in some area, and the individual is diagnosed with a disease. Sometimes the disease is life-threatening, and sometimes it isn't. But it all begins with a thought that is a lie from Satan's kingdom. Through thoughts that are sins against the spirit, over an extended period of time we can remove ourselves from God's protective covering and put our bodies at risk to disease.

Let me give you a true-life example. Delores Winder experienced a miraculous healing from an illness she'd had for over nineteen years. As a result, she launched a full-time healing ministry. She gives her testimony in her book, *Jesus Set Me Free.* I know of Mrs. Winder's credible ministry because she was a member of my dear Granny Carter's church in Arlington, Texas. My grandmother told me of how that church had prayed for her many times. In her book, she gives testimony of ministering to an elderly woman who was crippled with arthritis and was asking for prayer. As Mrs. Winder prayed for the woman, the Lord prompted her with the word "unforgiveness." As the story gradually unfolded, the woman revealed that she harbored bitterness toward her brother. He lived just two doors over, yet they had not spoken in more than twelve years (pp. 76-78). The sin of unforgiveness had changed this woman's body chemistry over an extended period of time, finally manifesting itself as a disease. In her situation, the disease was arthritis. The Lord revealed all this to her through Mrs. Winder.

Pastor Henry Wright of Pleasant Valley Church in Thomaston, Georgia, has also observed that simple arthritis, involving inflammation of the joints, is often a result of bitterness toward others (*A More Excellent Way*, p. 143). So here we have two ministers who specialize in a ministry to those with disease. They don't know each other and have written books seventeen years apart, and they have both come to the same conclusion about simple arthritis in the lives of these particular saints.

Now don't misunderstand my purpose. I am not arguing that we can track every disease to a specific sin. Unfortunately, I cannot offer any secrets to automatic healing. The spirit-mind-body connection is far too complex, with innumerable variables, for anyone to provide proof of a direct sin-to-disease relationship. I would argue that it doesn't matter if we have a sin-to-disease profile to begin with. It doesn't matter because there is no scriptural mandate for us to determine this connection.

Instead, we are commanded to sanctify ourselves wholly—body, soul, and spirit (2 Cor 7:1). That is what is important. We must maintain a proper relationship with our heavenly Father. When we do that, everything else falls into place. Our Father also commands us to confess our sins to one another so that we may be healed (James 5). Some in the body of Christ are empowered by the Holy Spirit to discern spirits. These saints can readily identify the sin issue without any knowledge of how or if the sin resulted in a disease. The sin issue is what is important, not the disease. The church, through the Word and through the Holy Spirit, is fully empowered to identify sin issues. Once those are resolved, the body has the opportunity to heal as God designed it to heal. Ideally, of course, sin issues should be resolved before disease ever occurs.

Another less common way that disease can be triggered is through trauma. We all carry hidden defects in our genes that we have inherited from our parents. Why is it that one person will develop a disease, when another person, even in the same family, does not develop the disease? Trauma causes this change and can occur at any time, even in the womb. Who is the author of trauma? Satan, of course. I previously mentioned a widower whose wife was diagnosed with multiple personalities. Her childhood was filled with horrific traumatic experiences that brought forth her condition.

"But seek ye first the kingdom of God and his righteousness; and all these things shall be added unto you" (Matt 6:33). In Matthew's gospel, Jesus compares the Kingdom of heaven to various things eleven times. But *what is* the kingdom of God? Paul states it plainly: "For the kingdom of God is not a matter of eating and drinking, but of righteousness, peace, and joy in the Holy Spirit" (Rom 14:17). In the context of disease, it seems that peace is very important. I'm not talking about the peace the world gives (John 14:27), but the peace that surpasses all comprehension (Phil 4:7)—a peace that is in the soul and which puts the body in a calm, healthy state.

Most of us are raised to accept subtle ungodly behavior, but we don't even know it. We seldom ask if our behavior is biblical. What we consider normal may not be acceptable in God's way of thinking. For example, we may be living with strife and conflict but calling it "peace," when the peace of God, according to His definition, is something altogether different. We have lost the true biblical meaning in our life. I had a conversation with a lady who was on staff at a church. She practically boasted that she had literally worried herself sick while her son was on a trip abroad. From her attitude, I don't think she saw her behavior as sinful. I don't think she connected her behavior, in worrying over her son, with Philippians 4:6: "Be anxious for nothing . . ." This means trusting your son to the Lord while he is out of the country. She was certainly missing out on the peace of God. At such times, we need the assistance of the mature believers of the church, those who have walked with the Lord and can tell us what it means to live with "righteousness, peace, and joy." They are the ones who have allowed

Christ to have greater and greater control in their lives. I am convinced that the sometimes overlooked invisible sins of fear, worry, and bitterness can, over time, contribute to disease.

In conclusion, Satan attacks our minds until he controls an area of thought. This process is so subtle that we don't see it happening, and it can take years. Such thoughts, both real and fantasy, can change the body's chemistry through the endocrine system, eventually causing disease. This occurs through the spirit-mind-body connection. Disease is not what God wants for us. He wants us to be in good health (3 John 1:2). We must always look to Him!

Chapter 6

A Biblical Response to Disease

One day in college, I was playing tennis with a Jewish friend. After our match, we had a friendly conversation that turned into a discussion of spiritual things. At one point, he said, "Well, I'm a Christian!"

His statement surprised me, so I asked, "How do you define 'a Christian'?"

"I'm a good person," he replied. "I'm nice and friendly, and I live a moral life."

I tell you this story so that there will be no misunderstanding. A person is not a Christian just because he or she lives according to Christian morality. This is a crucial issue. When we are born, we are spiritually dead, because we are part of a human race that is wicked. We do not meet God's standard of perfection. However, God loves us so much that He has provided a way to remove our wickedness and bring us to Himself. That's a lot of love! His way was the sacrificial death of His son, Jesus Christ, on the cross. When you believe in God and personally believe for yourself that Jesus' death is the reason to know God, then you become a Christian. You become alive spiritually and may have direct conversation with God. No priest, no rituals—just you and God, in the name of Jesus. If you haven't done this, then I encourage you to pray to God now and tell him that you have accepted the death of Jesus for yourself. He will be ecstatic to hear from you, and He will throw a party in heaven because of you!

Christianity is a unique religion, the only one in which God reaches down to mankind. Our relationship with God is based on belief only. The gods of the other major religions of the world do not reach down. According to their teachings, man must work his way to eternal fulfillment or heaven, and even then, after a life of work, they do not necessarily have a guarantee of acceptance by their god or eternal life after they die. Only in Christianity is eternal life given for belief alone as a free gift. This aspect of Christianity is relevant to disease, because without knowing God through Jesus Christ, we can never have victory over Satan and his kingdom. The name of Jesus is above all names, and His work on the cross is complete. It is His name and His work that give us victory over Satan and his kingdom. Otherwise, we are acting on our own authority, and alone, we will fail.

You or someone you love may be dealing with a disease that has come to you genetically, or, as I mentioned in chapter 2, through the sins of our ancestral fathers. Or perhaps you're dealing with a disease caused by the sins of others. Perhaps your disease originated with a sin issue that changed your health through the spirit-mind-body connection and the endocrine system. So what is the biblical response to disease? In my opinion, there is only one way for a Christian to deal with disease in his or her life, no matter the situation. You must sanctify yourself and immerse yourself in the Word of God and in prayer. There is no compromise. Our bodies are in position for optimal health when we are at peace with and have a right relationship with our heavenly Father. I also believe that we must examine our lives and open our private worlds to mature believers who will hold us accountable in a loving manner for sin issues in general, and for sins against the spirit in particular. A mature believer will not be afraid to speak the truth to us, even if it is hard to say. He/she will always maintain our privacy and confidentiality.

> *There is only one way for a Christian to deal with disease. You must immerse yourself in the Word of God and in prayer. There is no compromise.*

It's true that people who don't even know God are healed of disease, because our bodies are designed to heal naturally. Satan can work miracles of healing as well. But that does not change the biblical commands to the saint who is walking with Christ. We must still obey and follow the commands of our Father in heaven and sanctify ourselves.

About a month after Teresa was diagnosed, while we were attending church, the pastor read Ephesians 5:25: "Husbands, love your wives just as Christ also loved the church and gave Himself up for her." Later that day, I felt compelled to read further: "So that He might sanctify her, having cleansed her by the washing of water with the word." Right then, I decided I wanted to sanctify my wife and cleanse her with God's Word. I bought a one-year Bible, and on October 29, 2001, I started reading it to her. I read out loud almost every night. I finished fourteen months later, on January 27, 2003. It was one of the most loving experiences of our marriage. It gave us peace and strength and filled our minds with thoughts of God's goodness, love, and sovereignty over our lives. So husbands, I challenge you: Sanctify your wife. Make her holy before the Lord, according to Ephesians 5:25-26. Read God's Word to her every day, out loud. It will take a commitment, but it will be most rewarding and worth every minute of your time.

I also purchased the Bible on CD. There were times when we listened closely, and times when we would just let it play. We also purchased a few audiotapes from different ministries that we found most helpful, which included testimonies and healing Scriptures. From time to time, we would sit and listen to them and just absorb the truth of God. Then, when we received bad news from the doctor, we were prepared in advance. We would remember and personalize a verse such as Psalm 112:7: "Klay and Teresa will have no fear of bad news. Our hearts are steadfast, trusting in the Lord." Or Philippians 4:19: "My God shall supply all your needs, Klay and Teresa, according to His riches in glory in Christ Jesus."

When I was a teenager, I was convinced that my parents were set on taking all the fun out of my life that they possibly could. As soon as I had a great idea, like buying a motorcycle, the answer was, "No." I wanted a rifle like the guys on television, and the answer was, "No." What about a fast sports car? "No, no, no." I got a Volkswagen Beetle. It wasn't until I became a father that I understood that instructions (or rules, guidelines, directives) could serve several good purposes, including protection. I also realized that they brought blessings. When I lived by my father's rules, I got to live in his nice house, where my expenses were lower and I could put more money toward recreational activities. God's Word is similar. It is there to protect us and to bring blessings when we are obedient.

There is much debate in our day and age over the applicability of Deuteronomy 28 in its presentation of blessings and curses. Does keeping God's Word really bring blessings? Does violation of God's Word really bring curses? We can extend this debate a little further into the world of "Prosperity Theology." This is the belief that if you give $100 to the church, you will receive $1,000 in your checking account in the near future. I don't agree with either of these arguments, primarily because their proponents have changed the definition of blessings to refer to worldly and material things, instead of biblical and spiritual blessings. Let me explain.

A few months after Teresa died, our eight-year-old son made a remarkably profound statement. I find it amazing how a child can simplify some of the most complex issues. He said, "Dad, I know what they use for money in heaven!"

"Well, what is that?" I asked.

"Love," he answered. "Love in heaven is the same as money here. You just give love!"

Wow, what a great statement! The Holy Spirit had been speaking to his young heart. God is less concerned with *how much* money we have and more concerned with *what we do* with the money he has already given us—i.e., he is more concerned about our stewardship. If we change the claims of "Prosperity Theology" to say that when I give $100 to the church, I am going to receive a reward based on spiritual values, such as love, either in this life or in heaven, then I accept that line of thought. If the blessing and curses of Deuteronomy 28 are defined in spiritual terms, such as righteousness, joy, and peace, or the fruits of the spirit, then I can agree with that line of argument, too. However, I disagree with those who believe that material possessions will be the blessing. God simply doesn't place value on big-screen televisions or exotic vacations.

So how does all this relate to disease? If we keep God's commands, then in general terms we will receive his protection and blessings of health in our life. We are therefore much less likely to acquire a disease caused by our own sins against the spirit. So sanctify yourself. Don't be anxious or bitter, don't have self-hatred, and don't compare yourself to others. Be grateful and enjoy life and all that our heavenly Father has given us. All of these biblical commands have physical benefits as well as spiritual, and when we obey them, we are not causing unwanted chemical reactions in our bodies that will eventually put our health at risk.

I have taken time to encourage you to read the Word of God. In case this is new to you, then I'd like to give you a few verses that describe God's Word, which will provide you with a solid understanding of why you need to read, memorize, and speak God's Word. The Bible is not an ordinary book.

The apostle John writes, "In the beginning was the Word and the Word was with God and the Word was God. He was with God in the beginning" (John 1.1). At the end of the New Testament, John writes, "Then I saw heaven open, and a white horse was standing there . . . . He was clothed with a robe dipped in blood, and his title was 'The Word of God'" (Rev 19:11, 13). These statements serve as bookends for all creation, the beginning and the end. Jesus *is* the Word. Don't think for one minute that the Word of God is mere printed words on a page. The Word of God is Christ manifest.

> *For the word of God is living and active and sharper than any two-edged sword, and piercing as far as the division of soul and spirit, of both joints and marrow, and able to judge the thoughts and intentions of the heart.*
>
> *And there is no creature hidden from His sight, but all things are open and laid bare to the eyes of Him with whom we have to do.* (Hebrews 4:12-13, NASB)

This is a powerful statement. The Word of God is living and active.

> *So will My word be which goes forth from My mouth; It will not return to Me empty, without accomplishing what I desire, and without succeeding in the matter for which I sent it.* (Isaiah 55:11, NASB)

We must speak words of faith. This might sound unnecessary, but it's important for us to speak God's Word and pray God's Word *out loud.* Our adversaries in Satan's kingdom cannot read our minds. It's important that you speak out loud so that all of those around you, both seen and unseen, can hear your words of faith and belief in God's Word. This is not a "Name it, claim it" theology that some subscribe to. All our words of faith are still subject to God's plan. I spoke words of healing over Teresa every day, and the Lord still took her home because it served His purpose. Nevertheless, it is essential that you speak God's Word out loud.

Here is a healing verse from God's word:

> *He sent His word and healed them, and delivered them from their destructions.* (Psalm 107:20, NASB)

God's Word stands forever; it will never pass away (Matt 24:35, Mark 13:31 and Isaiah 40:8). Do you want to know the most effective way to pray? You must pray God's Word back to him. God cannot deny His own Word, so if you ask for grace or mercy, He will give you grace and mercy. If you ask for wisdom, He will give you wisdom, because He has already promised it in His word. Jesus quoted this Scripture to Satan when He was tempted:

> *He humbled you and let you be hungry, and fed you with manna which you did not know, nor did your fathers know, that He might make you understand that man does not live by bread alone, but man lives by everything that proceeds out of the mouth of the LORD.* (Deuteronomy 8:3, NASB)

The whole of Psalm 119 communicates the completeness of God's Word to us. It tells us that the result of being a doer of the Word is purity (v. 9) and that through the Word we will receive protection and strength (vv. 17-32). Additionally, we will receive wisdom (vv. 97-104), have guidance, "for the Word is a light to my feet" (v. 105), and finally that we will enjoy peace when we meditate on the Word of God (v. 165).

There are many, many verses on the meaning and power of God's Word, which tells us truth and cancels the lies that Satan and this world have told us. The Word renews our minds. Of course, none of this will occur unless you are reading and praying over God's Word. Our health and healing are in direct relation to the time we spend in prayer and in His Word.

Chapter 7

Helping Those Touched by Disease

If I were required to choose one word to describe a ministry to those with disease, I would choose the word *availability*. A synonym to this term might be *yielded*. All too often, we become subtly self-centered and begin thinking of how we're going to do this or that for the Lord. We've planned out just how it ought to be. Then things don't go as we planned. Many times, it's because we are not necessarily led by the Lord as much as by our own plan. I know about having my own plan. I am a reformed Type A personality and have been driven much of my life. Yet now I must admit to making mistakes that have taught me the difference between having goals and being driven, versus being led by the Lord and the Holy Spirit.

The prophet Isaiah captured the correct attitude of availability at the beginning of his ministry when he said, "Here am I. Send me!" (Isaiah 6:8). His heart was completely available and yielded to the Lord, and he did not have his own agenda. Mary demonstrated the same attitude in her response to learning of her impending pregnancy. She faced extreme social ridicule, if not stoning, yet she said, "Behold, the bond slave of the Lord; may it be done to me according to your word" (Luke 1:38). It was this same yielded availability that Jesus demonstrated in the garden of Gethsemane. Before His arrest, he prayed three times, "Father, if you are willing, remove this cup from me; yet not my will, but Yours be done" (Matthew 26:39, 42 and 44, NASB).

I think our heavenly Father directs the Holy Spirit to work on the inside of an individual. He starts in the heart and in a place that is beyond our reach. My first thought when I begin to minister to someone with a disease is that I can talk all day, but if the person's heart is not ready to hear, then I am wasting my breath. Are they at the point where they are ready to listen? Most people do not want to hear what the Bible has to say about disease, sin, or Satan's work in their lives. Their hearts are not ready. We certainly can't help someone who does not want help. Remember the old adage, "You can lead a horse to water, but you can't make him drink."

Sometimes we misapply our desire to help, and then it backfires and results in a casualty. Let me explain. Sometimes Christians who are available can be overbearing in their approach and actually cause harm. I've seen it happen over and over again. I can give you a personal testimony of two well-intended Christian ladies who went to a lady who was terminally ill with ovarian cancer. They told her that she was sick because of a sin issue in her life and that she would be healed if she confessed her sin. This was one of the most absurd stories I had ever heard. Fortunately, the ill woman was a mature believer and was not offended. She already knew what the Lord was doing in her life and how to respond appropriately. But what if she had not known the Lord?

This doesn't happen just in ministering to those who are ill; it happens in all areas of ministry when a passionate saint forces himself on someone who doesn't share his view. The saint's efforts are actually offensive and result in a casualty, when a person becomes so bitter and defensive that, in the end, they are further from the Lord than when they began their encounter with the well-intended Christian. My friend Dave Burchett has written an excellent book on this subject titled, *When Bad Christians Happen to Good People.*

I simply don't believe that the Holy Spirit causes casualties or creates conflict. In contrast, the Holy Spirit is a gentle and loving comforter. The Holy Spirit is patient and kind. God's ways are perfect. He opens people's spiritual eyes and prepares their hearts. We are simply His tools. He can wait a lifetime for someone to open his or her heart, but of course we are impatient and want to see results today! No, the work of the Holy Spirit does not cause casualties. Many times the problem is that we as saints don't stop to listen to the Holy Spirit first, and we get in His way. I have memorized 2 Timothy 2:24, for it is filled with God's wisdom:

> *The Lord's bond-servant must not be quarrelsome, but be kind to all, able to teach, patient when wronged, with gentleness correcting those who are in opposition, if perhaps God may grant them repentance leading to the knowledge of the truth, and they may come to their senses and escape from the snare of the devil, having been held captive by him to do his will.* (NASV)

I am always available to tell my story to those who inquire. Typically, I will wait for a second or third question before I start a conversation. That way, I can see if the Holy Spirit has prepared someone's heart. Until then, people are just being polite. If I tell my story to ten people, I would guess that only one or two actually understand my message. So what is it about the one or two that's so different? After all, it's the same message. The difference is that the Holy Spirit has opened their spiritual eyes and ears to hear the message. It's not my words, but rather the Holy Spirit working in their life. My highest calling is to be available to my heavenly Father and to be sensitive to the leading of the Holy Spirit.

My highest calling is to be available to my heavenly Father and to be sensitive to the leading of the Holy Spirit.

If someone who is dealing with a disease does have an open heart, then I move forward in gentleness and love. Sometimes I can see that the Holy Spirit has prepared a person's heart, because they have read James 5 and have asked the elders to pray for them. Simple conversation is the first step in any ministry to someone dealing with a disease. A skilled listener can ask intelligent questions and gradually peel away the layers of issues until they reveal the core reason for disease. Do you remember the seven reasons I started with? If you are helping an eighty-two-year-old man with lung cancer, you will certainly respond differently than to the thirty-five-year-old woman diagnosed with fibromyalgia. In the first case, the Lord may be preparing him and his family for his passing. The other may be a complex situation involving multiple causes. In some cases, the Lord may use you to lead a person to restoration and healing. In other situations, you may serve as a source of comfort and support.

To determine the root cause, I think a few things must happen. First, the person must allow you into their private world. You must establish trust and confidence regarding private matters. This takes time, and in our culture, we are conditioned to getting what we want right now. You must not put a timeline on ministering to someone with a disease; it's all God's timing. I know of one pastor who ministered to a lady for over a year and a half before she began to make progress from her disease. Second, it may help to probe into the conflict areas of a person's life. You may find a conflict with a family member, whether past or present, or a conflict in the violation of a biblical principle, such as self-hatred, guilt, or unforgiveness, or a conflict with God the Father.

One of the spiritual gifts given to the body of Christ is the distinguishing of spirits (1 Cor 12:10). You will know the people with this gift in your church if you seek them out; they are the mature believers who display the fruits of the spirit in their lives. They are the best ones qualified to carry on this ministry. If it is determined that there is a sin issue—and again, this is not always the case—the person must bring about a change in their behavior so that their body can heal. This is usually a change from the heart, and it is the greatest of challenges. Change is not easy.

It is vitally important to recognize that there are many legal hazards in a ministry to those with disease. For example, if, in the process of talking with someone, you become suspicious that child abuse has occurred, then you are required to report it to the governmental authorities. This includes any child abuse, even if unrelated to the person with whom you are talking. If you fail to report it, you are guilty of a crime yourself and can potentially be sued in civil court. (You must know your own state's laws on these matters.)

Also, you cannot tell people what to do with their medications unless you are a licensed medical professional in your state. The best thing to do is to tell them to pray and ask the Lord themselves what He would have them do. Then they can tell you what they have decided. A third area of difficulty is the potential for inappropriate emotional and sexual involvement on the part of the participants. Husbands and wives make great ministry teams, yet as a general rule, two women should minister to a woman, and two men should minister to a man. We have all heard of numerous ministers who have had to resign because of misconduct in this area. One of the wisest pastors I have ever known always kept his door open when counseling women one-on-one. He also had the most trustworthy and godly secretary that you would ever find. She was constantly working to protect the integrity of that church, and she was mature enough to maintain the confidentiality of that pastor's counseling ministry.

Ministry to those with disease and deliverance from sin issues should not be turned into a show or publicity stunt. Ministry should be private and confidential.

Deliverance can occur in one of three ways. First, as John writes, "You shall know the truth, and the truth shall make you free" (John 8:32). If we believe that we are ugly, and then one day we hear the truth of God—that we are wonderfully and beautifully made—then we stop thinking of ourselves as ugly. We are free of that thought, because we have heard the truth. Second, James exhorts us to "Submit therefore to God. Resist the devil, and he will flee from you. Draw near to God, and he will draw near to you" (James 4:7-8). I pray this regularly. I pray it out loud! The third way is through the "casting out of demons" that Jesus and the disciples did regularly.

No one wants to be labeled as a fanatic and lose his or her credibility, and too often people jump to extremes in their thinking. When it comes to dealing with Satan's presence in my life, I appreciate the words written by Neil T. Anderson in his excellent best-selling book, *The Bondage Breaker*. He recognizes the difference between a "power encounter" and a "truth encounter." It's not necessary to shout or scream at a person who is under Satan's oppression. It's not necessary to hit or make someone fall to the ground, or to show any type of power. These are scare tactics. When addressing an evil spirit, you merely speak biblical truth. Satan's agents can hear you just fine, and what they need to be reminded of is your authority as a child of Christ. As a minister, you have God's Word to stand on. You should be fully knowledgeable of Ephesians 6.

Scriptures are not specific on the details of Satan's work or how to identify those who are spiritually oppressed. I believe the Holy Spirit will empower you and lead you if He wants you there. You can also be attentive to some fundamental modes of communication. Watch others' body language, listen to what they say, and observe their behavior. Do they demonstrate the fruits of the spirit, or the fruits of the flesh? A Christian who is spiritually oppressed is a person who is not at peace. He/she demonstrates compulsive behavior in an area of life and does not listen to reason. This behavior occurs in different degrees, so don't expect to hear a person hiss like a snake. Most spiritual oppression is very subtle. But again, the most obvious evidence flows right out of the mouth. Yes, we all experience oppression on some level; this is part of our life's journey. But those who have a disease because of fear or bitterness or another sin against the spirit will reveal themselves in time through conversation.

In conclusion, opinions differ on how to proceed after a root cause is identified. I don't think there is a guaranteed formula or step-by-step process, because we are talking about matters of the heart and about a personal God. Some people find freedom in the privacy of their prayer closet, while others find freedom through the help of others. Some people have a disease that is not related to sin at all, while others do have sin issues but are spiritually blinded and unwilling to confess them or take responsibility for them. Some people come to a point of understanding their disease from a spiritual perspective and are healed. There is a full range of responses.

I recommend that you seek the Lord with all your heart and immerse yourself in His Word. Swim in his Word daily, and give your heart to the Lord. It will transform your life.

I was greatly encouraged by the book *Waking the Dead* by John Eldredge. In chapter 10, he makes recommendations on how to find freedom and successfully fight our daily spiritual battle. I won't repeat the whole chapter here, but it begins with a prayer in which we choose to abide in Christ. He then recommends several prayers that reconnect us with our Heavenly Father, as well as prayers to resist Satan.

I also encourage you to look at the books previously mentioned, *The Bondage Breaker* by Neil Anderson, *A More Excellent Way* by Pastor Henry Wright, and the others on my recommended reading list. Then prayerfully allow the Lord to lead you.

In November 2003, about four months before her death, Teresa called me into our home office to talk to me. She was clearly emotionally moved, which was unusual for her because she had a very calm and peaceful temperament. She told me that earlier that day while driving to the mall, an indescribable feeling had come over her. I asked her to describe it, and she said it was a "feeling of wholeness: body, soul, and spirit." She said she felt a freedom and a peace that she had not experienced since she was baptized. When she told me this, tears welled up in her eyes, and she wept. I didn't know how to respond, other than to tell her that the Holy Spirit had touched her to strengthen her. From that day on, her physical health declined, but her spirit was free. She never spoke one word of complaint. During the final months of her life, she thought mostly of the kids and me. Her love was rich, and we savored every moment. She kissed me every day and told me she loved me the morning before she fell into a coma. By God's grace, it did not last long, and she died later that night.

I have accepted that the Lord wanted to take her home before I was finished with her. I am grateful for having received such a wonderful and special love. It was the love of my heavenly Father flowing through the beautiful woman, whom He gave to me for a season and it came with the "the peace of God that passes understanding" (Philippians 4:7).

In closing, "I pray that in all respects you may prosper and be in good health, just as your soul prospers" (3 John 2, NASB). I pray that you place your hope in the Lord and "Set your mind on things above" (Colossians 3:2). Then you should be able to live in peace irregardless of your circumstance. The Lord will take care of the rest.

About the Author

Klay Rogers lives in Garland, Texas, and is a self-employed Certified Public Accountant and business broker. He has a business degree from the University of Texas in Austin, and has completed graduate work at Dallas Theological Seminary. He has been a Christian since childhood, and enjoyed sixteen wonderful years of marriage to his late wife Teresa. Klay is the parent of three busy kids and enjoys writing humorous country songs and spending time at the lake. He can be contacted through his website at www.KlayRogersCPA.com. He is available to do the Lord's work by giving testimony and teaching upon invitation.

Recommended Reading

Anderson, Neil T. *The Bondage Breaker.* 2nd ed. Eugene, OR: Harvest House Publishers, 2000.

Balch, Phyllis A., and James F. Balch, M.D. *Prescription for Nutritional Healing.* 3rd ed. Garden City Park, N.Y.: Avery Publishing Group.

Burchett, Dave. *When Bad Christians Happen to Good People.* Colorado Springs, CO: Waterbrook Press, 2002.

Capps, Charles. *The Tongue: A Creative Force.* Tulsa, OK: Harrison House, 1976.

Colbert, Don, M.D. *Deadly Emotions.* Nashville, TN: Thomas Nelson Publishers, 2003.

Craichey, K.C. *Super Health, 7 Golden Keys to Unlock Lifelong Vitality.* Minneapolis, MN, 2005

Eldredge, John. *Waking the Dead.* Nashville, TN. Thomas Nelson Publishers, 2003.

Hagee, John. *The Power to Heal.* San Antonio, TX: John Hagee Ministries, 1991.

McMillen S.I., M.D., and David E. Stern, M.D. *None of these Diseases.* 3rd ed. Grand Rapids, MI.: Revell Books, 2000.

Sapolsky, Robert M. *Why Zebras Don't Get Ulcers.* 3rd ed. New York, N.Y.: Owl Books, 2004.

SELYE, HANS, M.D. *The Stress of Life.* 2nd ed. New York, N.Y.: McGraw-Hill Companies, Inc., 1978.

STRONG, JAMES. *The New Strong's Expanded Exhaustive Concordance of the Bible.* Nashville, TN: Thomas Nelson Publishers, 2001.

TALBOTT, SHAWN. *The Cortisol Connection.* Alameda, CA: Hunter House, 2002.

WALFORD, ROY, M.D. *Beyond the 120 Year Diet: How to Double Your Vital Years.* Rev. and exp. Ed. New York, N.Y.: Four Walls Eight Windows, 2000.

WINDER, DELORES WITH BILL KEITH. *Jesus Set Me Free.* Rev. ed. Shreveport, LA: Fellowship Foundation, Inc., 2000. (The publisher may be contacted directly at P.O. Box 19370, Shreveport, LA, 71149-0370, 318-635-6728).

WRIGHT, HENRY. *A More Excellent Way.* Thomaston, GA: Pleasant Valley Publications, 2003.